WHAT'S YOUR PROBLEM?

WHAT'S YOUR PROBLEM?

KAREN DOCKREY

VICTOR BOOKS®
A DIVISION OF SCRIPTURE PRESS PUBLICATIONS INC.
USA CANADA ENGLAND

All Bible quotations, unless otherwise indicated, are from the *Holy Bible, New International Version,* © 1973, 1978, 1984, International Bible Society. Used by permission of Zondervan Bible Publishers.

Library of Congress Catalog Card Number: 87-81024
ISBN: 0-89693-381-4

CONTENTS

WHAT'S YOUR PROBLEM? addresses problems young teens face and helps them find God's solutions. They'll learn how to cope with their own problems, help friends who have problems, and wrestle with tough problems that trouble us all. As part of the Young Teen Feedback Elective series, this book presents creative Bible studies that will keep your young teens interested and challenge them to spiritual growth.

HOW TO USE YOUNG TEEN FEEDBACK ELECTIVES

You'll discover that these studies are especially geared toward young teens—a group in the midst of change. As they struggle to make the transition from children to adults, young teens sometimes show extremes of behavior—energetic one minute, withdrawn the next. These fast-paced studies offer a variety of teaching methods to appeal to sometimes hard-to-interest group members. Yet each creative session is firmly founded on the Word of God.

Each lesson focuses on one or more Bible truths that can be applied directly to young teens' lives. Make sure you have enough Bibles so that students who forget theirs can borrow them. Try to have some modern-speech translations on hand for easy comprehension.

If you're unfamiliar with Young Teen Feedback Electives, take a few minutes to study this overview of your elective study.

Flexible Format
Notice that you can study the topic of this book over a 12-week quarter. In addition, each subtopic is complete in itself, so you can also study part of this elective for four weeks, returning to the other studies at a later time. This format gives you flexibility to suit your program to the particular needs of your young people. It also lets you tailor the study to your schedule.

Introductory Page
Each session has an easy-to-use summary of the lesson on the first page to help you see the lesson at a glance.

- *Key Concept* clearly states the lesson's theme.
- *Meeting the Need* outlines general concerns and questions young teens have on the session's subject. By understanding their concerns, you can better help teens apply the lesson.
- *Session Goals* includes the objectives of the lesson in measurable terms. Each goal helps communicate the Key Concept and should be achieved by group members by the end of the session.
- *Special Preparation* gives you a checklist of what you'll need to lead the session.

Building the Body
The first minutes of each session are devoted to relationship building. These exercises, activities, and optional "warm-ups" will help your group get to know one another and you—a key to an open group where good communication can take place. These activities also provide a transition

time which takes young teens away from outside concerns and points them toward the group study.

Launching the Lesson
This section offers focus discussions and activities that zero in on needs and interests that will be covered by the Bible study later in the lesson.

Exploring the Word
This part of the study contains creative ways to communicate Bible truths and concepts. It not only helps *you* share God's Word, but it also allows young teens to discover God's Word for themselves.

Applying the Truth
This application section summarizes Bible truths and concepts. It helps young teens relate Christian faith and values to their everyday lives, answering the question, "What does this mean to me?"

Workout Sheets
These activity sheets encourage young teens to discover concepts, facts, and ideas in a variety of ways. The sheets are meant to be reproduced. Just tear out the master copy and make as many duplicates as you need. You may want to provide folders for group members to collect and save their Workout Sheets.

Student Books
Student books are available to help bring home Bible truths to young teens in your group. These lively books are written by men and women who know how to communicate to your young people. They can be used many different ways:

- Have group members read the chapter *after* each session so material covered in class will be reinforced and "come alive" at home.
- Have group members read a chapter *before* each session to stimulate their thinking on the subject and get them ready for in-class discussions.
- Use portions of the books *during* the group study. For instance, incorporate a case study from the book into a group discussion.

You can complete this elective study without using the student books, but we recommend them as an excellent tool to give students their own version of the material you study together. It's something permanent that they can refer to long after the group study has ended. These books are entertaining, informative, and fun to use. Their small size makes them portable; they fit easily into pockets or purses. Look for them at your local Christian bookstore, and add them to this elective study.

Before Each Lesson
Pray for your young teens as they work through this study. Ask the Lord to help you create an open atmosphere in your group, so that teens will feel free to share with each other and you.

After Each Lesson
Evaluate each session as you ask yourself the following questions: Did each student achieve the lesson goals? Why or why not? Did you have the right amount of time to complete the lesson? How many group members actively took part in the session? Are interpersonal relationships being nurtured in the group? How well did you prepare the lesson? How might you change your presentation next time?

WHAT'S MY PROBLEM?

PART ONE

Because many young teens find it difficult to talk about their deepest problems, this section gives them opportunity to examine these problems in a comfortable way. The sessions focus on:

- Understanding feelings
- Recognizing and resisting temptation
- Listening to loneliness
- Dealing with depression

As group members understand such problems as doubt, anger, jealousy, temptation, guilt, loneliness, and depression, they'll more easily find solutions that work. Help them recognize that their problems are normal and solvable.

The teaching methods used in this book encourage involvement. They are designed to make learning enjoyable and meaningful. You will help teens discover truth for themselves and thus better understand and know how to apply that truth.

Several of the sessions suggest more activities than you may have time to do in your session. This allows you to choose what works best for you. If one teaching approach does not appeal to you or meet your students' needs (and you know them best), you will still have enough material to fill the session. Even though you may not use all the material, prepare for all or most of it in case you have extra time.

Help your group members find out they can . . .
- Understand and grow through their feelings
- Tackle temptation
- Make the most of alone time and reach out to others
- Defeat depression

Their problems can become tools for growth, rather than just sources of frustration. Together you'll learn that God cares about the problems we face and goes through them with us, helping us find the answers.

WHAT'S MY PROBLEM?

SESSION 1

HOW IT FEELS UNDER THE PROBLEM PILE (Selected passages)

KEY CONCEPT

We can respond to doubt, anger, and jealousy in ways that strengthen our faith, solve the problem, and make us more secure.

MEETING THE NEED

This session will respond to the following student concerns:
- "Why am I the only one who seems to have problems?"
- "I don't understand myself sometimes."
- "If I were a better Christian, I wouldn't struggle with negative emotions."

SESSION GOALS

You will help each group member
1. memorize several problem-solving strategies,
2. identify some misconceptions about doubt, anger, and jealousy,
3. create three-step plans for handling doubt, anger, and jealousy.

SPECIAL PREPARATION

_____ Bring extra Bibles, small and large paper, masking tape, pencils, and markers.
_____ Duplicate Workout Sheets #1 and #2.
_____ Write the problem-solving strategies for "Draw Me a Picture."

BUILDING THE BODY

WORKOUT SHEET

Divide the group into teams of four. Distribute copies of Workout Sheet #1, "Share Sheet," and direct them to fill it out privately. After a moment or two, direct the foursomes to share their answers, one question at a time (each member shares his answer to question 1, then each shares for question 2, and so on). Circulate among the groups to encourage them and answer questions.

After most groups are finished, ask: **Was it easier to share what you like or what you don't like about yourselves? What you do well or poorly?** Emphasize that God created us and it is fine, though sometimes hard, to notice our good qualities. Say: **When you notice the good in yourself, you recognize God's handiwork.**

Ask: **What problems did you write?** Point out the similarities in problems. Emphasize: **Most youth struggle with problems similar to yours.** Ask: **Which of you had problems that you hesitated to write or didn't write down at all? I simply want you to raise your hand, not tell the problem.** Explain: **These four sessions will examine some of the problems we find hard to talk about: doubt, anger, jealousy, temptation, guilt, loneliness, and depression.**

Ask: **What difference does it make that Jesus became a man and felt emotions as we do?** (He knows how to handle feelings; He's the only one who can truly say, "I know just how you feel." He's a great source of answers!)

Emphasize: **The bad news is that problems are here to stay. Christians at all stages of maturity struggle with problems. But the good news is that Jesus has the answers. Together we'll discover and implement some of His answers in these sessions.**

LAUNCHING THE LESSON

DRAW ME A PICTURE

Before the session write these problem-solving strategies on separate pieces of paper and place them in a paper sack:

TALK TO A FRIEND
WRITE OUT YOUR FEELINGS
TALK TO AN ADULT YOU TRUST
PRAY, TALKING WITH GOD ABOUT WHAT TO DO
FIND BIBLE VERSES ADDRESSING THE PROBLEM
ASK QUESTIONS TO UNDERSTAND THE PROBLEM BETTER
GIVE IT SOME TIME
LIST PROS AND CONS OF EACH OPTION
THINK THROUGH CONSEQUENCES
ASK, WHAT WOULD JESUS DO?

To memorize these problem-solving strategies, play drawing charades. Divide youth into teams of four and direct each team to number off, 1–4. Give each team paper and pencils and explain these directions: **In this game we will get an overview of some effective personal problem-solving strategies. Person #1 from each team will come to me and look at the skill. Then he will return to his team and draw it for them. He may not talk, use letters, or use numbers. When your team guesses correctly, send your person #1 back to me. The first person #1 back wins a point for his team. Then person #2 takes a turn, and so on. Any questions?** Explain that teams don't have to guess word-for-word—the general idea is close enough.

Call for persons #1. Pull a problem-solving strategy out of your bag and show it to all four at once. Say "go" when all have seen it. Repeat until all helping skills have been drawn and guessed. (If teams have trouble guessing the abstract ideas, change the rules to allow for words that are not part of the wording given on the item being drawn.)

Say: **Without realizing it you have worked on memorizing 10 problem-solving skills. Who can name all 10?** Let several volunteers try it. Congratulate everyone who tries. Challenge youth: **Seek to notice every time we use one of these skills in this session and work on developing them in your own lives.**

FOCUS ON FEELINGS

Explain: **Many of our problems produce or start with feelings that we don't know what to do about. Three big ones are doubt, anger, and jealousy. During this session we'll examine why we feel these feelings, how they can help us grow, and what we can do about them.**

Divide into three teams. One neutral way to do this is by shoe color or style. Notice three variations among your group's shoes, such as all tennis shoes become the "Doubting Group," all black or brown shoes become the "Angry Group," and all colored shoes become the "Jealous Group." Explain: **Each of you has an emotion to examine. Once you understand it you will teach the other two groups what to do when they feel that way. You will stay in these groups for the rest of the session.**

Direct the groups: **Write a statement a person might make who is feeling your group's emotion. We'll use our discoveries to solve this situation later in the session.**

Examples:

Doubt—"Does God really exist? I used to think so, but I just don't see any evidence of Him." "I'm an atheist. That God stuff makes no sense."
Anger—"I got in trouble for something I didn't do!" "How could she treat me that way?"
Jealousy—"He won the election instead of me!" "She went out with him when she *knew* I liked him."

Student book option: Rather than writing their own situations, let youth use the situations of Jim, Pam, and Linda in chapter 1 of the student book.

EXPLORING THE WORD

WORKOUT SHEET

Distribute Workout Sheet #2, "Find the Mistake." Direct the groups to complete the section dealing with their emotion. Corrected statements are below with comments in parentheses:

DEALING WITH DOUBT

1. When Jesus' disciples had trouble believing, He asked them why, gave them evidences that He was alive, and opened their minds so they could understand the Scriptures (Luke 24:36-39, 45). (When we doubt, Jesus helps us understand why, answers our questions, gives us evidences, and helps us understand the evidences and the Bible.)
2. Jesus gave them evidence to strengthen their faith: He let them see His pierced hands and feet, asked them to touch Him to see that He actually had flesh and bones, ate to show He was alive, and explained the Scriptures about Himself (Luke 24:36-49). (Rather than criticize us when we doubt, Jesus helps us understand the firm truth of His existence.)
3. Thomas said that unless he put his finger where the nail marks were and put his hand into Jesus' side, he would not believe it (John 20:24-25). (It is fine to ask for evidence for our faith. Many people have joined and been harmed by weird cults simply because they refused to investigate the cult's beliefs and were told "just believe." One of the best characteristics of Christianity is that it stands firm. The more you ask, the more you see how real Jesus is.)
4. Jesus gave Thomas the evidence he needed to believe (John 20:24-29). (Jesus wants to help us deal with doubt. He always has the answer we need. We never have to fear questioning our faith because the answer will be, Yes, God definitely exists and loves you!)
5. Thomas said, "My Lord and my God!" (John 20:27-28). (Thomas understood who Jesus was and responded with faith. Our efforts to deal with doubt usually deepen our faith, not weaken it.)

ANSWERING ANGER

1. All Christians get angry from time to time. We must handle our anger and not let our anger lead to sin (Ephesians 4:26). (Anger can be good or bad, depending on why we feel it and how we respond to it. An example of anger leading to good: anger over mistreatment of a friend leads to stopping that treatment. God gets angry and His anger leads to good.)
2. Settle your anger the same day you feel it (Ephesians 4:26). (Not letting the sun go down on your anger assures that you settle the problem rather than stewing over it and making it worse.)
3. Holding anger in can give the devil a foothold (Ephesians 4:27). (Our anger can be used by the devil to lead to greater evil. Unresolved anger leads to depression, aggression, grudges, broken friendships, murder, etc.)
4. We are to get rid of anger when we feel it (Colossians 3:8). (We can do this by recognizing it and talking it out with God or a friend.)
5. Jesus got angry about the Pharisees' stubborn hearts (Mark 3:5). (Jesus' anger led to positive action. Other verses indicate that God also got angry about His people's lack of faith and obedience.)

JOLTING JEALOUSY

1. God is a jealous God, especially when His people worship other gods (Joshua 24:19). (God's jealousy is designed to draw us back to Him, to encourage us to live His way, because only His way brings happiness to us. His jealousy is holy and righteous, not like ours which is selfish and vengeful.)
2. Jealousy is as unyielding as death (Song of Songs 8:6). (Because it is closely connected with love and because it is so strong, jealousy is hard to handle. Trust in the other's care is one of the most effective fighters against jealousy.)
3. True love does not include jealousy (1 Corinthians 13:4-7). (Trust and jealousy are opposites. Jealousy usually comes because we fear the other doesn't like us as much as someone else. Reassurance, expressions of love, and lots of talking can replace destructive jealousy with security.)
4. The disciples were angry (and probably jealous) because they wanted positions of honor too (Mark 10:35-41). (Anger and jealousy often go hand in hand. Recognizing that you wanted what someone else had can help you get over the feelings. Work toward positive competition, rather than winning at all costs. Once again, the more secure you feel, the less likely you'll be prey to competitive jealousy.)
5. Jesus said that those who want to become great must be servants (Mark 10:42-45). (One cure for jealousy is to find and meet the needs of others. When you concentrate on others you don't have time to worry about whether you're getting your "fair share.")

After youth have found the mistakes, call on each group to point out the mistakes in its section. Suggest that the other two groups note the mistakes as each group reports. Supplement with the above comments and then reemphasize the following points:

1. **Doubt, anger, and jealousy are not necessarily sins. They can lead to sin, but they are not sins in themselves. But be careful—check to see why you feel angry or jealous; if it's selfish, it's wrong.**
2. **Because God experienced anger and jealousy, we know they have some positive element. He felt those feelings when His righteousness was being violated, not out of selfishness.**
3. **God offers help, not condemnation, when we experience doubt, anger, and jealousy. But He wants us to work through these feelings and go on.**
4. **Responding to doubt, anger, and jealousy directly can make us stronger, more secure, and happier.**

Emphasize: **The Bible always has the answers we need.** Call on someone to read Philippians 4:13. Ask: **Whose power do we have for handling problems?** (Jesus'.) Explain: **Jesus not only has the answers, He has the power to help us handle the emotions that trouble us.**

APPLYING THE TRUTH

STRATEGY

Guide youth to develop a three-step strategy that they think God would recommend for solving problems. Give these instructions: **Using the Bible**

truths you have discovered, create a three-step strategy for facing your group's emotion.

NOTE: Because they have to come up with their own strategies, your youth may find this procedure difficult. Give substantial encouragement and ideas when needed. Explain: **Though it may be hard to come up with a plan, it gives you practice for coming up with real life plans. That's usually not easy either. Thinking through what you would do makes it easier to handle these emotions when they come to you (and they come to every Christian at least once!).** As you guide them, encourage their ideas and suggest one point at a time from the following sample plans if necessary. Even if you give the whole plan to youth step by step, they will have worked with you to find it, and will remember it.

Sample strategies for the three emotions are:

Doubt

1. Find the reason for your doubt. ("The teacher asked, 'Why do you believe in God? We know there's no proof for His existence.' ")
2. Take your doubt to God. ("God, they say you don't exist. I wonder if you really do. . . . ")
3. Find the solution to your doubt. ("I talked to Marcie and she helped me discover evidences for God's existence, such as the goodness in people, the sense of right and wrong we all have, and the archeological proofs of the accuracy of the Bible. I'm glad to know the God I've always believed in is really real.")

Anger

1. Recognize your anger. ("I get so mad when Edward brags.")
2. Discover the reason for your anger. ("I feel like he thinks the rest of us aren't as good as he is.")
3. Find a solution to your anger. ("I could do three or four things: I could ask God to help me feel more secure so Edward couldn't make me feel so dumb; I could compliment Edward so he wouldn't feel the need to brag; I could get it out by telling Mom how much it bugs me.")

Jealousy

1. Admit that you feel jealous. ("I thought I just didn't like the new girl. I think I'm actually jealous.")
2. Ask God why you feel jealous. ("God helped me realize that I fear my friend will like the new girl better than me.")
3. Replace jealousy with greater security. (Tell your friend, "I'm feeling jealous of the new girl because I'm afraid you'll like her better than me. I know my feelings are unreasonable and that she needs friends too, but I just need reassurance that you still care about me.")

Post the strategies on the wall or bulletin board.

SOLVE YOUR OWN PROBLEMS

Redistribute the problems youth wrote under "Focus on Feelings." Call for each group to read its problem and for all three groups to suggest ways to solve the problems based on the Bible study and the three-step plans. Point out: **Another group's three-step plan may offer tips useful for addressing your emotion.**

SHARE SHEET

Take a few minutes by yourself to fill out this sheet. Then share your answers with your small group.

1. One thing I like about myself:

2. One thing I don't like about myself:

3. One problem I have:

4. Two things I do well:
   1.
   2.

5. Two things I do poorly:
   1.
   2.

FIND THE MISTAKE

Each statement has a mistake. Read the Bible verses to find the mistake, and write in the correction.

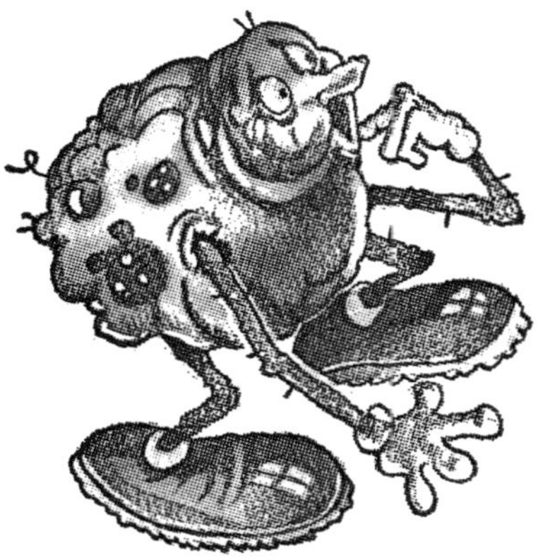

DEALING WITH DOUBT

1. When Jesus' disciples had trouble believing He had really been raised from the dead, He told them they didn't have enough faith (Luke 24:36-39, 45).
2. Jesus said that if they couldn't believe without evidence, no amount of evidence would convince them (Luke 24:36-39, 45).
3. Thomas had not been with the disciples at Jesus' first appearance to them, but he believed what they said about Jesus (John 20:24-25).
4. Jesus appeared to Thomas a week later and scolded him for doubting (John 20:24-29).
5. When Jesus told Thomas to put his finger in His hands and his hand into His side, Thomas said, "OK" (John 20:27-28).

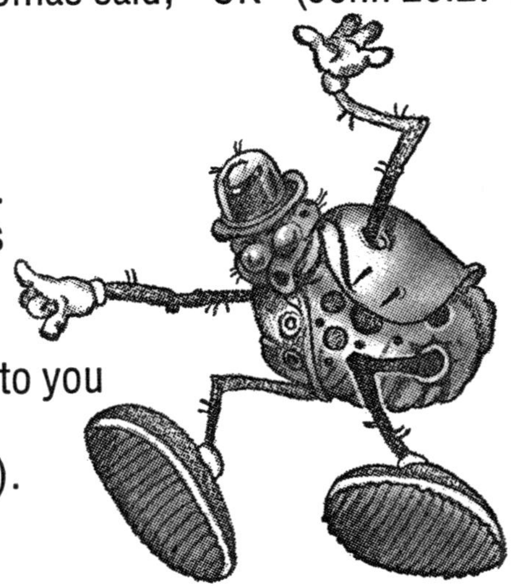

ANSWERING ANGER

1. A good Christian will never feel angry (Ephesians 4:26).
2. Wait until you feel like it to settle your anger (Ephesians 4:26).
3. It doesn't hurt to keep anger inside (Ephesians 4:27).
4. There's nothing you can do about anger once it comes to you (Colossians 3:8).
5. Jesus never got angry, so neither should we (Mark 3:5).

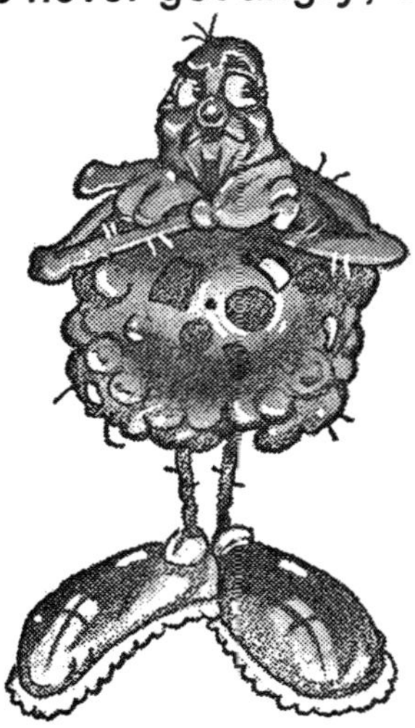

JOLTING JEALOUSY

1. God never felt jealous (Joshua 24:19).
2. Jealousy lets go easily (Song of Songs 8:6).
3. True love always includes a measure of jealousy (1 Corinthians 13:4-7).
4. The disciples were pleased with James and John when they asked for places of honor (Mark 10:35-41).
5. Jesus said when they became great they could have servants (Mark 10:42-45).

SESSION 2

TACKLING TEMPTATION (Selected passages)

KEY CONCEPT

Temptation can lead to sin, but it is not a sin in itself.

MEETING THE NEED

This session will respond to the following student comments:

- "If God knew what I thought about, He wouldn't be very happy."
- "Am I bad if I'm tempted?"
- "I thought the Christian life was easier! All I've had is trouble since I became a Christian."

SESSION GOALS

You will help each group member

1. list temptations teens face,
2. discover ways Jesus fought temptation,
3. practice fighting temptations.

SPECIAL PREPARATION

_____ Bring extra Bibles, pencils, markers, large and small paper, masking tape, and chalk.

_____ Consider talking with one or two group members who will share a 30- to 60-second testimony for "Talking with Jesus."

_____ Duplicate Workout Sheets #3 and #4.

BUILDING THE BODY

BEST AND WORST

Call for each person to share: **What were the best and worst things about your day? Each of us will share our best and worst. Who would like to begin?** Start with yourself or a volunteer and proceed clockwise around the circle. Encourage hesitant teens to share by giving them time (10 seconds seems like an eternity of silence) and expressing warmhearted interest.

Follow up the sharing time by pointing out one or both of these points:

1. **Where you hurt matters to me and when you are happy, I feel happy.**
2. **Sometimes we feel that nothing good ever happens to us. Each of you have shared at least one good thing in your day. Let the good help you get through the bad.**

Explain: **One of the bad things in our lives is temptation. It's hard to know how to respond to it! Be assured of one thing: facing temptation doesn't make you bad. Giving in is the sin, not the desire to give in. In this session, we hope to discover just why temptation has so much power over us and practice some strategies for resisting it.**

LAUNCHING THE LESSON

TEMPTATION TALK

Challenge the boys to compete against the girls to write as many temptations as they can. Position the teams as far apart as your meeting space permits and give them large paper and markers. Say: **I'll give you 60 seconds to write more temptations than the other side. Make most of them temptations that youth face. Wait until I say "go." Any questions?** Pause to answer questions. Then say, "Go!" Circulate between the teams to encourage and give ideas. When 60 seconds have passed, call time and direct the groups to tape their lists to the wall. Call on teams to alternate calling out one temptation at a time. Discuss the lists using such questions as:

1. **How do the lists differ?**
2. **How are they the same?**
3. **Which of these temptations are unique to youth?**
4. **Which are easiest to fight? Hardest?**
5. **Which present more severe consequences when someone gives in to them?**

WE'VE ALL GOT IT BAD

Call on someone to read 1 Corinthians 10:13. Discuss the verse using these questions: **Does anyone have a unique temptation?** (No.) **Why can't we say, "I couldn't help myself; it was just too great a temptation for me"?** (Because God won't let us be tempted beyond what we can bear.) **What will God do for us when we're tempted?** (Provide a way out so we can stand up to the temptation.)

Ask: **If God has promised never to let us be tempted beyond what we can bear and promises a way out of the temptation, why do so many people give in to temptation?** (We don't *really* believe that God's way will make us happy; wrong seems more fun than right; we get ourselves into difficult situations; we fear people will laugh at us if we resist; we want to give in more than we want to resist; we don't ask for God's help; some of us aren't Christians; we don't know that we don't have to give in; we rebel against God; we let the feeling of the moment take over.)

Explain: **The best protection against temptation is a close relationship with God. When we trust Him to make us happy, we'll believe Him when He says that wrong will make us sad. Then we work harder to resist temptation.**

TALKING WITH JESUS

Point out: **In order to have a strong relationship with God, you have to have started a relationship with Him. We call this "becoming a Christian." Who would like to explain how they became a Christian?** Encourage Christian group members to share briefly how and why they received Christ.

Supplement testimonies with: **Becoming a Christian means giving your life to Jesus. You notice that no thing or person has been able to make you really happy. You realize that you've done wrong and need forgiveness. You believe that Jesus loves you so much that He died for you. You accept Jesus' forgiveness and love for you. You rejoice that Jesus now sees you as justified, "just as if I'd never sinned." You have a fresh start and a constant companion in life. Jesus gives you love, wisdom, help for problems, strength, security, and more.**

Instruct youth to bow their heads as you guide them in prayer. Explain: **I will introduce topics. I want you to concentrate on each topic and feel free to pray out loud or silently. Your prayers can be words, phrases, or sentences.** Pray along with youth but, to keep from stifling their opportunities to pray, pray no more than a couple sentences and allow 10 full seconds of silence before you speak.

- **Begin by telling God why you're glad to be a Christian or why you think you'd like being a Christian.**
- **Thank Jesus for His qualities, like constant love and understanding our temptations.**
- **Confess wrongs that are on your mind. Perhaps you have hurt someone or have failed to obey God in an area.**
- **If you are not a Christian, take this opportunity to invite Jesus into your life. Know that once you ask Him, He is in your life to stay.**
- **Finally, tell God anything else that is on your mind.**

Thank your group for their openness and their honesty. Explain: **You can**

tell God whatever you feel, think, and need. You who have become Christians during this time, let me know so I can rejoice with you and help you grow. You've made the most important decision of your life. You who are still thinking, bring me your questions or talk to another Christian you trust. Keep asking until you understand. You won't want to miss the adventure of life with Jesus.

EXPLORING THE WORD

WORKOUT SHEET

Emphasize: **It's important to realize that even the best Christians with the closest relationships struggle against temptation. In fact, sometimes the stronger you are, the harder the devil works on you. Jesus Himself was tempted, as we'll examine in our Bible study. Temptation is never a sin. Giving in to it is the sin.**

To discover the strategies used by the devil and the ways Jesus combated them, guide youth: **Complete the crossword puzzle on Workout Sheet #3.** Add interest by allowing them to work in pairs and challenging them to see who can finish the puzzle first. Explain that the crossword puzzle is based on Matthew 4:1-11 from the *New International Version.*

Key:

ACROSS	DOWN
4. JESUS	1. FORTY
6. LORD YOUR GOD	2. BREAD
7. ANGELS	3. FASTING
12. SPLENDOR	5. MOUNTAIN
13. STONES	8. SON
14. DEVIL	9. SPIRIT
16. WRITTEN	10. WORSHIP
	11. WORD
	15. AWAY

When they have finished, check answers by reviewing the temptation of Jesus with comments similar to these:

The Holy (9 down) led Jesus into the desert to be tempted. God doesn't tempt people. The (14 across) does. Jesus was hungry after (3 down) 40 days and 40 nights. The devil dared Jesus to prove He was the (8 down) of God by telling the (13 across) to become bread. Jesus responded to the devil by quoting the Bible. He said, "It is (16 across), 'Man does not live on (2 down) alone, but on every (11 down) that comes from the mouth of God.'" The devil then responded by using the same religious words (4 across) used: "It is written." The devil quoted the Bible accurately, but he used it the wrong way. He said, "He will command His (7 across) concerning you, and they will lift you up in their hands." Jesus recognized that the devil had misused Scripture, and He quickly responded with the better verse for the situation: "Do not put the (6 across) to the test." Then the devil took Jesus to a very high (5 down) and showed Him all the kingdoms of the world and their (12 across). He promised all this to (4 across) if He would worship the devil. Jesus told the devil to just get (15 down) and then quoted Scripture again: "(10 down) the (6 across), and serve Him only." The devil had focused on the splendor, the obvious attractive features of the kingdoms. Jesus saw through him and did what was right. After the temptation, the (7 across) attended Jesus.

Discuss the puzzle using questions like these:

- **Which of the devil's strategies does he seem to use most often with you?** (Manipulating your need; daring you; misusing Scripture; showing the splendor of the temptations; and more.)
- **The devil first attacked Jesus in His area of greatest pain: hunger. Around what needs or hurts does he seem to focus his attacks on teenagers?** (Need for a boyfriend or girlfriend; wanting to be popular; needing friends; wanting independence; wanting something now.)
- **How did Jesus resist the devil's temptation strategies?** (Recognized his lies; quoted Scripture; told him to get away; told the truth.)

QUOTE THE BOOK

Explain: **The Bible verses Jesus quoted were from the Old Testament Book of Deuteronomy.** Ask: **What Bible verses do you tend to depend on when you are tempted?** (Their sharing may be sparse due to shyness or lack of knowledge.) Call on a youth to read Hebrews 2:17-18. Ask: **How do you feel knowing that Jesus has been through temptation too? How does this make Him better able to help you through your temptations? Think about the temptation that torments you most right now. What advice do you think Jesus would give you for handling it?** (Can be private response.)

STUDENT BOOK OPTION

If you have the student book, direct youth to find the section called "The Devil's Tricks." Challenge each: **Choose one illusion and tell a way the devil might use that illusion on you or someone you know.** (Example: "He might offer me an attractive but false solution by telling me that if I just drink a little I'll get invited to more parties. That may make it seem like I have more friends, but I'll really just be making a fool of myself.")

APPLYING THE TRUTH

LET GUILT BE GOOD

Ask: **How do you know if you are being tempted?** (Feel guilty; realize you want to do wrong.) **Did you know that some guilt isn't real guilt? The devil uses it to frustrate us. For example, many youth feel it's their fault when their parents divorce. That's not good guilt because it's false. Also the devil often keeps us feeling guilty after we've been forgiven. That's not good guilt either.**

How do you know if the guilt you feel is good guilt or bad guilt? (Good guilt agrees with the Bible; bad guilt stays after you've been forgiven. Good guilt motivates you to find the wrong and make it right; bad guilt makes you feel guilty for doing something which is really OK.) Emphasize: **All the guilt**

you feel indicates the need for attention. You either need to recognize that you don't need to feel bad for false guilt or you need to seek forgiveness for real guilt. Talk with God and Christians you trust.

Tell two stories of guilt based on Matthew 26–27 and John 21:15-19: **Two men in the Bible, apparently due to social pressure, betrayed Jesus. Judas turned Him over to the authorities and Peter denied knowing Him. What did Judas do when he realized his sin?** (He tried to give back the money he took for betraying Jesus and then hanged himself.) **What did Peter do when he realized his sin?** (He wept bitterly and later accepted Jesus' forgiveness and went on to become a church leader.) Emphasize: **Guilt is designed to lead us toward right, not condemn us for life. Don't make Judas' mistakes and condemn yourself. Accept Jesus' forgiveness and then move on to doing right as Peter did. The next few minutes we'll discover some ways to do so.**

IT DOESN'T BOTHER ME!

Direct group members: **Choose one temptation from the posters that tempts you and one that you have no trouble resisting.** Discuss these using such questions as: **What makes it easy to resist the temptation that doesn't bother you?** (Encourage specific ideas such as "Beer tastes bad to me.") **What makes the hard-to-resist temptation hard to resist?** (Encourage specific responses again.)

Suggest that each listen to others who found their hard-to-resist temptation easy to resist. Explain: **All of us find it easy to resist certain temptations and find others hard. We can encourage each other by sharing strategies that work for us. Realize that the devil won't bother you in an area easy for you to resist. Feel encouraged that you're doing well in some areas and transfer the resisting skills you use to harder areas. Let's practice for the next few minutes.**

Give each youth a piece of paper, a pencil, and these instructions: **Pretend you are the devil. Write a tempting letter using some of the strategies he used in Matthew 4:1-11. Choose one of the temptations on the posters you made near the beginning of this session or make up your own. Make your letter so tempting that no youth could resist.**

Collect the letters and shuffle them. Direct group members to choose one of the letters and to defeat the tempting strategies in the letter using the guidelines on Workout Sheet #4, "Resisting Temptation." Ask: **With what words or actions would you resist the temptation in your letter? Work as a group to resist as many temptations as time allows.**

Close by emphasizing: **Temptation and guilt are not sins in themselves; rather, they alert us to an area that needs spiritual attention.** Write RUN vertically on the chalkboard and overview this strategy to fight temptation:

Realize what tempts you and run from it
Understand the devil's schemes and how to fight them
K**N**ow that resisting temptation can make you stronger and happier

CROSSWORD DISCOVERIES

WORKOUT SHEET # 3

To discover the strategies used by the devil to tempt Jesus and the ways Jesus resisted them, complete this crossword puzzle. You'll find the answers in Matthew 4:1-11 (NIV).

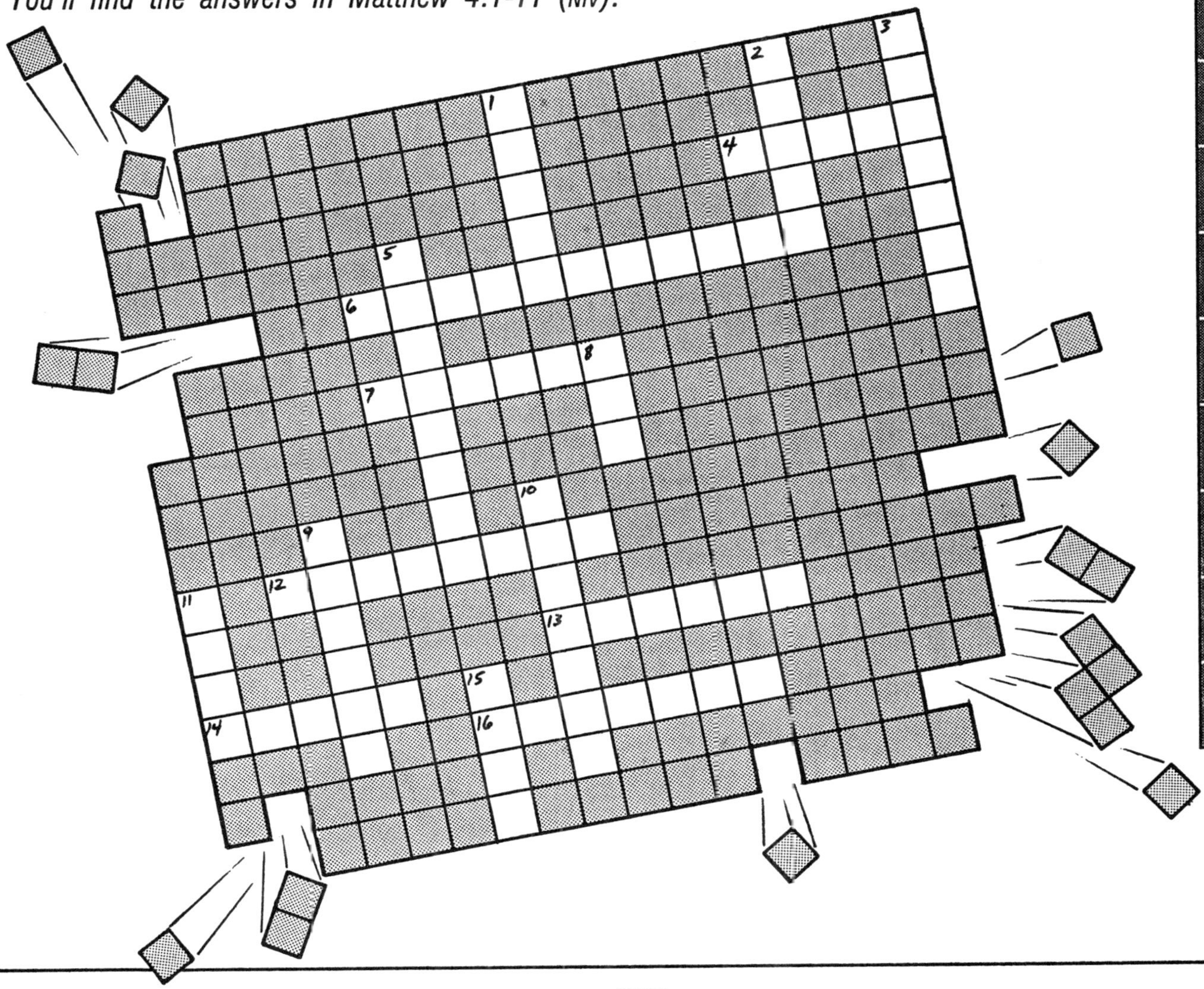

ACROSS

4. The devil used the same religious words ______ used: "It is written."

6. Jesus recognized that the devil had misused Scripture, and He quickly responded with the better verse for the situation: "Do not put the ______ to the test."

7. The devil quoted the Bible accurately, but he used it the wrong way. He said, "He will command His ______ concerning you, and they will lift you up in their hands."

12. The devil emphasized the ______ of the kingdoms.

13. The devil dared Jesus to prove He was the (8 down) of God by telling the ______ to become bread.

14. God doesn't tempt people. The ______ does.

16. Jesus responded to the devil by quoting the Bible: "It is ______."

DOWN

1. Jesus had been fasting this number of days.

2. "Man does not live on ______ alone, but on every (11 down) that comes from the mouth of God.

3. Jesus was hungry after ______.

5. Then the devil took Him to a very high ______.

8. The devil dared Jesus to prove He was the ______ of God by telling the (13 across) to become bread.

9. The Holy ______ led Jesus into the desert to be tempted by the devil.

10. Jesus quoted Scripture again: "______ the (6 across), and serve Him only."

11. (See 2 down.)

15. Jesus told the devil to just get ______.

RESISTING TEMPTATION

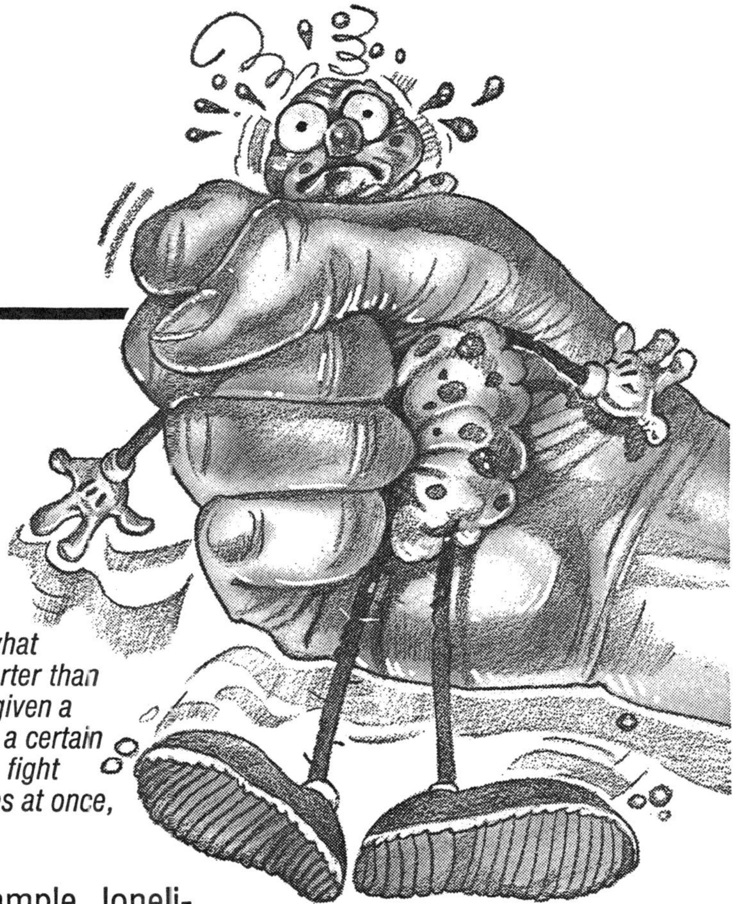

The devil *is a master at knowing just what tempts you and just how to get you to give in. Be even smarter than he is by noticing and knocking his schemes. You have been given a tempting letter that is written to make you want to give in to a certain sin. Based on that temptation, use the strategies below to fight the devil's schemes. (Because he doesn't use all his schemes at once, you won't be able to answer every guideline.)*

What weakness is the devil attacking? (For example, loneliness, uncertainty, etc.)

Point out the truth the devil left out.

Correct the half-truths you find.

Circle lies the devil used.

With what words does the devil speak for God, but say what God wouldn't say?

How does the devil misuse the Bible?

WHAT'S MY PROBLEM?

SESSION 3

ALONE BUT NOT LONELY (1 Kings 19:1-18)

KEY CONCEPT

Loneliness usually comes for a specific reason. Recognizing that reason can help us fight it.

MEETING THE NEED

This session will respond to the following student comments:
- "Nobody likes me."
- "I feel lonely in a crowd."
- "I'm the only one at home on a Saturday night."

SESSION GOALS

You will help each group member
1. discover reasons for loneliness,
2. illustrate Elijah's experience with loneliness,
3. discern helpful from harmful loneliness fighters.

SPECIAL PREPARATION

_____ Bring extra Bibles, pencils, markers, large and small paper, masking tape, and chalk.
_____ Arrange the chairs in one large circle and put a piece of paper and pencil in each chair.
_____ Duplicate Workout Sheets #5 and #6.
_____ Bring a song for the "Evaluating Our Music" option. Bring a tape or record player that projects well.
_____ Bring paper plates with eye holes cut out.

BUILDING THE BODY

WHY I LIKE YOU

Give each group member a sheet of paper on which he is to write his name across the top and leave it in his chair. Say: **Stand, move one chair to the left, and write a compliment to the person whose name is on the paper in that chair. Repeat until all of you have written a compliment on each paper.** Emphasize that the comments must be positive, that they do not have to sign their names to the compliments, and that they can write the compliments in all directions (upside down, diagonally, etc). Suggest: **If you do not know the person well, compliment something about her appearance, such as, "You always have a smile for everyone," or "You look very nice in blue." Be as specific as possible.**

When everyone has made it all around the circle, direct them to sit in their own chairs and read their compliment sheets.

Discuss: **How do you feel after reading your compliment sheet?** (They will probably share a range of feelings, such as good, great, happy, not sure whether to believe it or not.) **Do you have trouble believing or accepting any of the compliments? Why?** (Youth may share something like this: "I can't believe this one. I'm not that good," or "If this person really knew me, she wouldn't compliment me like this.") Emphasize: **All the compliments are true. The people who wrote them did so because they've seen those characteristics in you. Of course, no one is perfect, but you exhibit those characteristics at least some of the time.**

What would you think about getting this many compliments every day? (Would probably enjoy it.) **Why don't we compliment each other more often? Why do we seem to find it easier to cut down than to compliment?** (It seems safer and easier; giving compliments sometimes embarrasses people; other people cut down; we don't notice the good; we don't know how to compliment.)

Explain: **When no one tells us what we do well, we start to wonder if we ever do right or if anyone likes us. But when this many people compliment us, we feel secure, loved, and anything but lonely. As a group we can combat loneliness by pointing out the good we see in each other. We can help each other feel loved, understood, and needed.** Call on someone to read Hebrews 10:24-25. Comment: **We have just practiced this verse. Let's commit ourselves to doing it daily. If you will commit yourself to complimenting at least one person a day, raise your hand.** Smile encouragingly and then say: **Now let's explore some other causes for and solutions to loneliness.**

LAUNCHING THE LESSON

LONELINESS JOURNEY

Direct group members to get comfortable, sitting or lying on the floor if appropriate, and to close their eyes. Guide their thoughts with these questions, pausing for a few seconds between each:

Think for a moment about the last time you were lonely. (Keep your eyes closed.) Where were you? Who was with you, if anyone? What was this person doing or not doing? Did this person's actions ease or increase your loneliness? How?

If you were alone, what caused your loneliness? What event happened or did not happen? What did someone say or not say? Do or not do? Did you do something for which you feel ashamed? Were you frustrated? What was the reason?

What did you do about your loneliness? Sleep it off? Cry it out? Be depressed for awhile? Take it out on someone? Talk to someone? Pray? How did God or your friends help? What finally eased your loneliness? Were you pleased or frustrated with the way your loneliness ended? Did your actions help or hurt? What would you do differently next time?

You may open your eyes.

Say: **Let's jot down some of our thoughts about this and other times we felt lonely. We'll help each other learn from both the satisfying and frustrating parts of our past experiences.**

WORKOUT SHEET

Distribute Workout Sheet #5, "Listening to My Loneliness," and give these instructions: **Privately complete each sentence with your first thoughts. Though you'll have opportunity to share your responses, no one will be forced to share.**

Share responses to Workout Sheet #5 in groups of about six. If your group has ten or less, share in one large group. Give each team markers and two large pieces of paper labeled "Causes of Loneliness" and "Solutions to Loneliness." Give these instructions: **Share your responses to one question at a time. Jot down responses to sentences 1 and 4 on the "Causes" poster and responses to sentences 5 and 6 on the "Solutions" poster.**

Compliment the groups by pointing out their good work: **Your genuine sharing has enabled you to understand loneliness better. Together you have discovered some reasons for and possible solutions to loneliness. Now tape your posters to the wall.** Supplement their lists of reasons and solutions with these samples.

Reasons: I'm not included; some people make me feel inferior; I've done something which makes me feel bad; people don't like me; some people treat me like dirt and then I feel rejected and lonely; somebody who is hurting took it out on me; I'm sick and nobody comes to see me; my problem seems different than anyone else's; I'm afraid; I don't have enough money, ability, looks; nobody understands me; my best friend betrayed me; I'm afraid God has left me; I'm insecure; I blew it; my friend is moving away; I don't know how to get along with people.

Solutions: Go to a friend's house; focus on others; go to my room; talk with God; find time to pray; call a friend; talk it out with someone who will listen; find something interesting to do during alone time; go out with friends; find an activity and join it; wait it out; figure out why I'm lonely; learn to get along with people better; solve fights.

Ask: **What similarities did you discover among your answers?** (Possibilities: We all get lonely for similar reasons; my reasons for getting lonely are different than yours, but we feel the same feelings.) Emphasize: **There's always a reason for loneliness. Finding that reason is the first step toward solving it.** Return the group's attention to the lists of possible solutions. Ask: **Which of these help loneliness? Which might make it worse?** See the student book for more possible solutions.

EXPLORING THE WORD

SEE YOU IN THE COMICS

Divide group members into teams of about five. Direct the teams: **Create a comic strip that tells Elijah's story in 1 Kings 19:1-18. Break the passage up into parts, and each of you draw one or two frames of the comic strip. Write at the bottom of the frame the verses illustrated. Add dialogue in your own words. For example, for verse 2 Jezebel's messenger might say, "Jezebel promised that by tomorrow you'll be dead too!" Stick figures are fine. In fact, that's what I'd draw! When the frames are finished, tape them together and hang them on the wall. Paper, markers, and tape are here on the table.**

Circulate and encourage the teams. If teams are struggling, suggest these divisions for the cartoon frames:

Frame #1: vv. 1-2 (or can be two frames)
Frame #2: v. 3
Frame #3: vv. 4-5a
Frame #4: vv. 5b-7
Frame #5: vv. 8-10
Frame #6: v. 11a
Frame #7: v. 11b
Frame #8: v. 12a
Frame #9: vv. 12b-14
Frame #10: vv. 15-18

Now that teams have discovered the facts through their cartoon research, discuss the passage using these questions: **What situations led up to Elijah's loneliness?** (Exhaustion after a big spiritual event—God sent fire to burn up the sacrifice [chapter 18]; threat by Jezebel; feeling like he was the only one who believed; all the other prophets had been killed.) **How did he deal with it?** (Ran; said he'd had enough; complained to God; wanted to die; went to sleep.) **How did God help him conquer his loneliness?** (Met his physical needs for sleep and food; listened to him both before and after he slept; spoke to him quietly; gave him companions to help with the work load—Hazael, Jehu, and Elisha.)

Point out: **Elijah was not only lonely—he was depressed. Often the two**

go hand in hand. In the next session we'll examine depression and how to respond to it.

APPLYING THE TRUTH

Try this optional exercise to benefit a group which particularly enjoys music.

EVALUATING OUR MUSIC

Prior to the session enlist someone to bring a tape or record, depending on your playing equipment, of a currently popular song that deals with loneliness. Write out the words of the song on a large sheet of paper, or have the group do this.

Play the song and encourage everyone to sing along using the written words as a guide. Analyze the song using these questions as a guide: **What does this song say about loneliness?** (Examples: I'm lonely without you; I'll never be lonely again; stay so I won't be lonely tonight.) **What is its solution to loneliness?** (Common negative solutions in secular songs are: dwell on the loneliness; go to bed with your boyfriend or girlfriend; find a sweetheart no matter what the cost; look to romantic love; commit suicide. Common positive solutions are: focus on others' needs; talk about it; find something to do with your alone time; realize loneliness comes to everyone occasionally.) **What solution would God offer in this situation?** (Possibilities: tell Him about your feelings; find the unmet need and meet it; spend time with a good friend; write out your feelings.)

After you've listened to the song, ask: **Why do we listen to music when we're lonely?** (To cheer ourselves up; to feel more blue; to hear someone else who feels sad too.) **When is listening to music helpful?** (When it helps us understand and conquer our loneliness.) **When is listening to music harmful?** (When it makes us more blue; when it gives us false solutions.) Ask: **What songs help you with loneliness?** (Whatever they listen to.) Explain: **Our favorite songs reflect how we feel and what we think we should do about it. As you listen to music, recognize which solutions work and which are false or temporary. Then choose to listen to songs that remind you how to solve loneliness rather than make it worse.**

TAKING OFF OUR MASKS

Say: **Raise your hand if you have ever felt lonely but let no one know.** Explain: **Rather than hiding when we have loneliness, let's find a way out.** Pass out paper plates with eyes cut out of them. **On the outside of this mask, write or draw ways you hide your loneliness. On the inside, draw words and actions you can use to let a friend help you with loneliness.**

When the masks are finished, call for volunteers to share the actions they put on the inside. (Possible answers: "I'm lonely because Bill is out of town. Can we do something together this weekend?" tell a friend; call on the phone; write a letter about your feelings; cry; ask a friend about her problem.)

Assure your group: **There is nothing wrong with feeling lonely. But you don't have to let it go on. Like other uncomfortable feelings, loneliness signals the need for action.**

WORKOUT SHEET

Distribute Workout Sheet #6, which contains a message to be decoded. (Correct answer: "Look not only to your own interests, but also to the interests of others.") After they have deciphered it, explain: **This is a portion of Philippians 2:4.** Instruct youth to write "Philippians 2:4" on their Workout Sheets, and pause while they do so. Continue: **This verse reminds us that one of the best ways to combat loneliness is to become involved in meeting the needs of others. When you forget yourself long enough to help someone else, your loneliness tends to take care of itself.**

AROUND WE GO

Step A: Challenge youth: **Starting with the person on my right, we'll go around the circle and state ways to be involved with each other's interests and needs. If you can't think of something within 10 seconds, you stand up. If you think of something the next round, you can sit back down.** (Samples: Listen; ask, "What's wrong?"; ask, "Would you like to talk?"; ask what they miss about the person they're lonely for; talk to everyone who walks in the room; be sure no one sits alone; invite everyone along; notice when someone is feeling lonely; be aware; encourage; share experiences; offer friendship; express sympathy; phone them.) Encourage as many different and specific responses as possible. Go around the circle two or three times (more, if ideas are still flowing).

Step B: Continue the same game but with a different assignment: **There won't always be someone around when you feel lonely. What if you're at home by yourself when loneliness strikes? Tell something interesting and productive you can do during lonely times to ease your own loneliness.** (Possibilities: Write letters; read; work on a hobby; do homework; watch a good movie; plan what you want to do next time you're with friends; work on your car; do something you enjoy; make a meal for your family; talk to a family member; read an article. The student book suggests more possibilities.)

Close by reading Psalm 34:18 and Jeremiah 29:11. Assure your group: **These Bible truths promise that we won't feel lonely forever and that happiness will return. God understands our loneliness and is ready and waiting to help. All we have to do is call on Him.**

WORKOUT SHEET # 5

LISTENING *to my Loneliness*

1 ■ I feel loneliest when . . .

2 ■ When I listen to a song about loneliness I . . .

3 ■ Some of these songs are . . .

4 ■ Sometimes a certain person does or says something to make me feel lonely. The words, actions, or characteristics of this person are . . .

5 ■ To try to escape my loneliness I . . .

6 ■ Loneliness leaves me when . . .

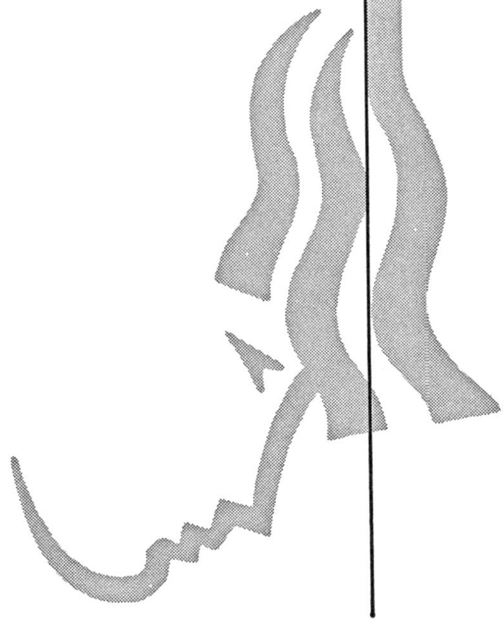

WORKOUT SHEET # 6

DECIPHER LONELINESS

Unscramble each word to discover the key to leaving loneliness behind:

kolo ont lyno ot ruoy now

____ ___ ____ __ ____ ___

setinrest, tub laso ot

_________ ___ ____ __

het setinrest fo

___ _________ __

tohres.

______

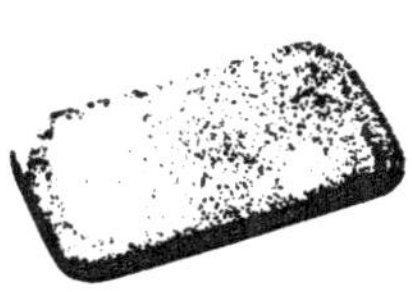

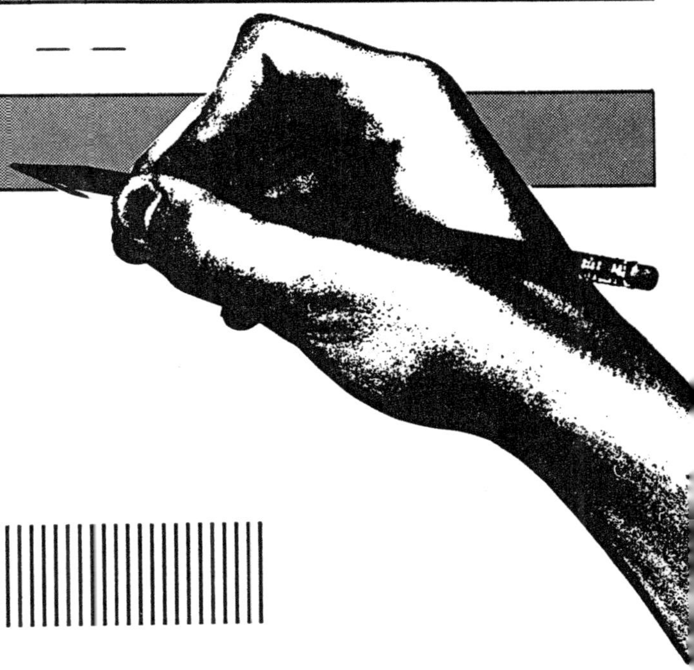

WHAT'S MY PROBLEM?

SESSION 4

DOWN ABOUT DEPRESSION (Psalm 32)

KEY CONCEPT

Depression alerts us to needs we have. Meeting the needs gets rid of the depression.

MEETING THE NEED

This session will respond to the following student concerns:

- "Is it a sin to be sad?"
- "I don't see why I should even try. I always mess up."
- "Nothing's wrong I'm just depressed."

SESSION GOALS

You will help each group member

1. discover causes for depression,
2. find out how unconfessed and confessed sin make us feel,
3. match solutions to causes of depression.

SPECIAL PREPARATION

_____ Bring extra Bibles, pencils, paper, and chalk.
_____ Duplicate Workout Sheets #7 and #8.
_____ Write words on cards for "Focus on the Word."

BUILDING THE BODY

TRUST WALK

Pair group members and designate one of each pair the "leader." Give these instructions: **Leaders, I'd like you to lead your partner on a walk. The boundaries are _______** (this room; this floor of the building). **Followers, you are to keep your eyes closed at all times during the walk. Leaders, earn and keep your partner's trust. Don't purposely run her into a wall or chair. It's crucial that you take good care of your partner.** The walk will last two minutes (shorter if your space is small).

After questions direct the couples to begin their walks. Observe but make no comment (unless one youth is endangering another!). When you call time and they return, debrief the experience using questions like these: **Leaders, how did you feel knowing your partner's safety was in your hands? Followers, how easy was it to trust and follow your leader? Did any of you open your eyes? Why? Followers, how did you know you could trust (or not trust) your leaders?**

Explain: **We all want the trust of our friends and we want them to trust us. One place to practice our trust is in helping each other with depression. We all feel sad from time to time and it helps to know someone will help us through it.**

WHOM DO YOU TRUST?

Call for each youth to tell about one person they would go to for help with a problem. It is not necessary that they mention the person's name, but encourage them to tell what it is about the person that makes him or her easy to trust. (Examples: Understands me; doesn't blab my problems to everyone; listens a lot; has good ideas for helping.)

LAUNCHING THE LESSON

STUDENT BOOK OPTION

If you have the student book, have someone read Rebekkah's story. Ask: **Why do you think Rebekkah is depressed?** Let several students share possibilities and then direct them to search the student book for the probable cause of her depression (fatigue, letdown after a big weekend). **Is depression a sin?** (No, it indicates a need that requires attention; it's a signal, not a sin.)

WORKOUT SHEET

Continue the search for causes of depression by saying: **Let's find more causes for depression. Circle the 10 causes hidden in the word**

search on Workout Sheet #7. You may work in pairs. As they work, play contemporary Christian music. It would be ideal if you could find songs that explain how God helps with sadness. (Youth can suggest some.)

Overview the answers: Horizontal–FAMILY AND FRIEND PROBLEMS; GUILT; REJECTION; ANGER; THREATENED SECURITY; DISAPPOINTMENT; LOSS; CHANGED RELATIONSHIP. Vertical–FAILURE; SPIRITUAL HIGH. Diagonal–ARGUMENTS; FATIGUE.

Discuss: **Were you surprised at any of the causes?** (Examples: Unresolved anger often shows itself as depression–when we hold anger in, we get sad. Guilt gets us down until we confess.) **Which causes seem a little confusing?** (Answer questions. Explain the two more general categories: "changed relationships" and "loss of security." The first involves such changes as divorce, breaking up, growing apart from a friend you used to be close to, you or a friend moves away, moving toward independence from parents, relationship problems, and more. Any time a relationship changes, especially to less closeness, depression can come. "Loss of security" is a feeling that the people and situations you had depended on won't, or might not, be there anymore. For example, you offend a friend and she doesn't like you anymore, or you're afraid that she won't. Both are hard.) **Which causes do you think affect youth most often?** (Youth are the authorities on this one! Examples: anger, disappointment.)

Explain: **Many of these causes can be real or imagined. For example, your security may be threatened because you really lose your friend or you just fear that you will. Either can make you depressed.**

HERE'S HOW WE SAY IT

Challenge group members: **I will read several statements. I'd like you to tell me the cause for depression which is behind each. Many situations have more than one cause.** (Or give one statement to each person and let them read the statements to the group.)

"I got cut from the team." (Disappointment.)
"My mom is mad at me again." (Family problems; argument.)
"I failed the test." (Disappointment; threatened security.)
"She won't like me anymore because of what I did." (Fear of changed relationship; threatened security.)
"I feel awful after practicing all day." (Fatigue.)
"Because of the accident, I'll never be able to walk again." (Loss.)
"Robbie broke up with me." (Changed relationship.)
"I'm furious with Kurt, but I dare not tell him." (Anger held in.)
"I shoplifted that backpack." (Guilt.)
"Kathie moved to another state. Who will I talk to?" (Loss.)
"When will they realize I'm old enough to make my own decisions?" (Family problems; changed relationship—moving toward independence.)
"My folks are divorcing." (Threatened security; disappointment; family problems; changed relationship.)
"My grandfather died." (Loss.)
"She's been criticizing me again." (Friendship problems.)

After these statements, challenge youth to give you a sad statement they or friends have made. With the group, identify the cause of the depression.

EXPLORING THE WORD

FOCUS ON THE WORD

Say: **Psalm 32 describes one of David's battles with depression. The first two verses describe how happy a person feels when all is right between him and the Lord. The next several speak of his feelings of depression, and the last verses share the joy he felt when he was forgiven and happy again. David's depression was caused by something he did wrong. Find your word in the psalm and study the verse(s) that use it to discover the role that word plays in depression.** (Give each person one of these words. Sample answers follow each.)

Blessed—vv. 1-2; how we feel after we've asked for and received forgiveness
Transgression—vv. 1, 5; going against God; a way to create depression
Forgive—vv. 1, 5; what God does when we confess; makes us feel good again
Sin—vv. 1-2, 5; doing what God forbids or not doing what He commands
The Lord—vv. 2, 10-11; He forgives, loves, and brings joy
Silent—v. 3; failure to confess sin; a way to hold sin inside; it creates depression
Bones—v. 3; what hurts when you're depressed
Groaning—v. 3; what you feel like doing when you're depressed
Hand—v. 4; God's hand; seems heavy when you're depressed
Strength—v. 4; what you have little of when you're depressed
Iniquity—v. 5; another word for "sin"; something you don't want to cover up
Confess—v. 5; doing this makes your guilt-caused depression go away
Hiding place—v. 7; what God provides for us when trouble comes
Teach—v. 8; God promises to do this so we won't be sad so often
Mule—v. 9; what we act like when we won't listen to God
Trust—v. 10; a way to avoid woes and experience God's love
Rejoice—v. 11; what you feel like doing when depression goes away

Help students find their verses and meanings. When most have found their word, walk through the passage with them using comments similar to the following. Encourage them to respond to questions about their words.

David wrote this psalm. He was depressed because he had done something wrong. Three words for "doing wrong" are *transgression, sin,* and *iniquity.* What verses use these words and what do they have to do with depression? (Verses 1-2, 5—When you do wrong and don't confess, you feel awful.) **David started out the psalm talking about being *blessed. Blessed* means happy. According to verses 1 and 2, what circumstances make you blessed?** (Transgressions forgiven, sins covered, sins the Lord does not count against him, spirit is no deceit.) **Who can put this in their own words?** (Example: God has *forgiven* me.)

How did David feel when he kept *silent* about his sin? (vv. 3-4) (Awful! His *bones* wasted away; he *groaned;* he felt like God's *hand* was on him; *strength* was sapped.) **Have you ever felt so sad that your body hurt? That you had no energy?** (Pause for response.) **Then you know what David went through. What did he decide to do about his problem?** (v. 5) (*Confess.*) **What did God do after David confessed?** (*Forgave* him.)

Then how did David feel? (Great!)

David's confidence and renewed joy in God is expressed through the rest of the psalm. His bout with depression taught him several things. If your word fills in the blank, stand and read it:

1. Even when the mighty waters rise (which means scary and threatening problems come), God is like a (hiding place) who protects us from troubles.
2. God will (teach) us the way to go and will give us good advice.
3. People who don't understand that God brings happiness are like a stubborn (mule).
4. When I (trust) God, I free Him to love me.
5. Having been helped through a tough time is something to (rejoice) about!

Close the discussion of the passage by asking: **What else might God teach you through a depressing experience?** (What to do next time; how important a certain person is to me; to trust Him and His Word.)

GOD AND ME

Explain: **One of the best things you can do when you're depressed is to talk with God like David did. Tell Him honestly every rotten feeling you're going through. Then, like He did with David, He'll guide you to a solution and back to happiness.**

Guide youth to write their own psalms to God. Offer three options:
A. Paraphrase Psalm 32:3-5.
B. Write a song to God about a time you were (or are) depressed.
C. Write a poem about trusting God in times of depression.

Provide paper, pencils, and encouragement.

When everyone is finished, call for volunteers to share their creations. Compliment something about each.

APPLYING THE TRUTH

CHARADE THE SOLUTIONS

Divide the group into teams of about six. Give each team 60 seconds to list actions that solve depression. Then say: **Now we'd like you to pantomime those solving actions. One team at a time will act out the action and the rest of us will try to guess. The team that guesses correctly will receive a point. We'll keep a list of the actions you portray here on the chalkboard.** Call for each team in turn to act out the solutions.

If you have student books, direct youth to search chapter 4 for solution ideas.

Sample solutions include: Take a nap; talk to a friend; eat something nourishing; list all the things that have gone well the past week; read Psalm

32 and other Bible passages that detail sad feelings that become happy; break the situation down into manageable parts; talk to an adult you trust; get professional help. (IMPORTANT: Don't limit the list to these. You and your group will have even more ideas.)

Emphasize: **We sometimes choose actions that can't solve depression. These seem good at first but only make it worse. Who can think of some faulty solutions to depression?** (Drugs, suicide, withdrawal, aggression, vandalism, drinking, sex, ignoring the feelings.) Ask: **Why do we feel like doing these things?** (We see no other way to solve the problem.)

Emphasize: **It's not wrong to *feel* like doing these things, but it is wrong to do them. When you feel like trying one of these faulty solutions, talk to someone you trust (even if it's just you and God) and find another solution. It's better to talk about destructive solutions than to try them. Then substitute a solution that works. You'll be glad you did.**

WORKOUT SHEET

Review the unit by reminding group members of three basic solve-your-own-problem strategies. Read the acrostic below: **ACT on your problem by spelling it out:**

- **A**dmit the problem. You only make problems worse when you ignore them.

- **C**ontact someone who can help. This may be God, a friend, an adult, or simply yourself. God can work through all of these sources. Just be sure the help you get is the help that really solves your problem.

- **T**ake the teaching to heart. Decide what God can teach you through the problem. Maybe He has shown you a way to avoid the problem in the future. Maybe you can now be more sensitive to someone else with the same problem. Maybe you have learned to trust His ways rather than ways that oppose them. Maybe you've discovered what really matters in life. Maybe you've learned that even when you don't understand, you can trust God to be in control.

Give each person a copy of Workout Sheet #8. Direct them: **Think about a problem you are currently facing. Write how you will A-C-T on it. This is private and no one will be asked to share. If you aren't sure where to start, I will be glad to help, or your first action might be to "ask someone to help you figure out what to do!"** While youth work, circulate and encourage. As they finish, instruct them to fold the papers and put them in their Bibles at Philippians 4:19.

Reemphasize: **Having problems does not mean you're bad or weird. It means you're human. Attack each problem as it comes and concentrate on the joy. Rather than letting problems get you down, A-C-T on them!**

Word Search

WORKOUT SHEET # 7

Find 12 causes of depression in this word search. Words are written horizontally, vertically, and diagonally. Some causes are two or three words together.

F	F	A	M	I	L	Y	A	N	D	F	R	I	E	N	D	P	R	O	B	L	E	M	S
A	K	I	G	U	I	L	T	J	O	P	Z	Y	F	L	O	R	T	C	M	L	O	R	P
I	H	I	M	O	M	R	E	J	E	C	T	I	O	N	Y	E	L	F	X	Y	R	T	I
L	R	A	Q	W	R	X	O	F	Z	E	B	R	A	A	Z	R	W	A	N	G	E	R	R
U	P	R	R	T	Y	U	C	B	A	I	L	O	V	E	U	J	E	S	U	S	X	X	I
R	X	M	T	G	T	Y	M	K	L	T	B	N	K	X	L	Y	U	E	M	C	I	Y	T
E	X	Y	X	D	U	Y	U	C	Z	Y	I	H	A	V	P	R	X	M	T	L	O	R	U
E	L	R	W	M	C	M	R	E	S	O	A	G	O	R	C	Z	I	M	M	S	L	I	A
M	M	C	O	Y	L	E	E	C	M	C	O	F	U	R	C	M	O	X	Y	A	M	C	L
C	M	I	L	C	Y	L	S	N	P	C	L	R	Y	E	P	C	L	R	C	M	L	Y	H
M	C	M	O	E	A	L	C	H	T	C	M	A	O	J	C	C	W	J	C	M	W	Y	I
T	H	R	E	A	T	E	N	E	D	S	E	C	U	R	I	T	Y	C	A	L	C	E	G
C	M	A	C	M	E	D	I	S	A	P	P	O	I	N	T	M	E	N	T	R	C	Y	H
L	O	S	S	R	C	H	A	N	G	E	D	R	E	L	A	T	I	O	N	S	H	I	P

Now jot down some specific things that get you depressed.

WORKOUT SHEET # 8

ACT ON IT

What's a problem that has you down? A-C-T on it using this prescription.

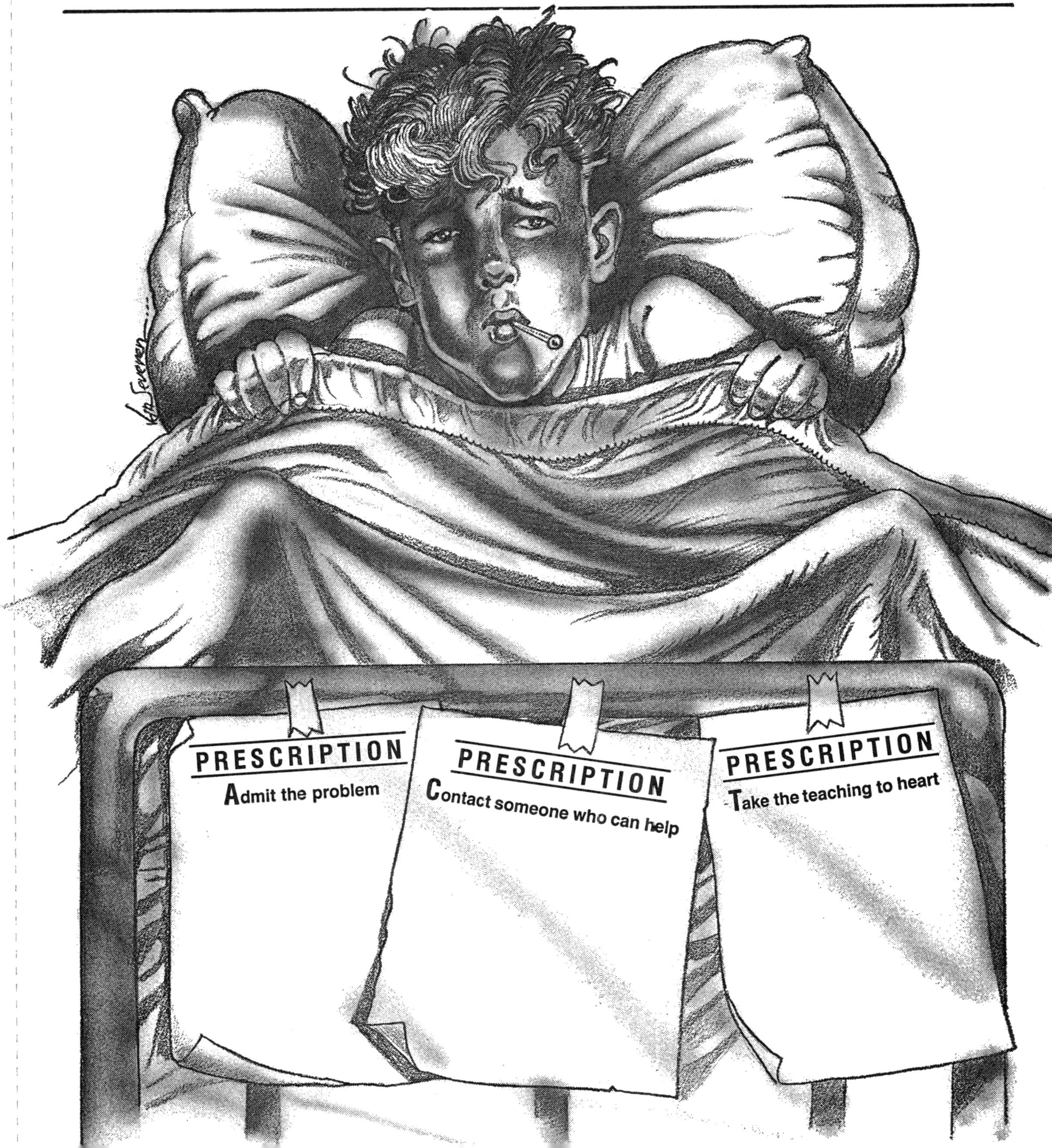

WHAT'S YOUR PROBLEM?

PART TWO

Young teens usually tell each other about their problems before they tell adults. That's why this section guides them in developing peer counseling skills. The four sessions focus on basic helping skills and the biblical basis for each. The skills are . . .

- Listening
- Choosing helpful words
- Giving good advice
- Finding adult help

Rather than simply reading about how to listen, choose helpful words, give good advice, and find adult help, your group will practice these skills. They'll discover both wrong ways and right ways to help through role plays and case studies and by solving their own real problems. They'll use guides, tried and true principles, and the best guide of all, the Bible.

Because the procedures are active, it may seem that you are entertaining your group rather than teaching them. But remember the principle of involvement: we learn better and remember longer what we are involved in. Bible truth makes a deeper impact on youth when they discover that truth for themselves. Resist the urge to sit them down and explain what every passage means. Instead, guide them to interact with God's Word and with each other to discover His truth. These procedures are designed to help you do this.

As you teach this unit, take care to communicate that helping with problems is one way to let God love a friend through you. Rather than following an easy formula, helping is loving people God's way with the words and actions He suggests. Encourage your students to practice applying the truths they discover both in class and outside of class, and to let you know how things go. Assure them of God's concern for their problems and the problems of their friends.

SESSION 5

IS ANYBODY LISTENING? (Selected passages)

KEY CONCEPT

When you listen to your friends you help them solve their problems.

MEETING THE NEED

This session will respond to the following student comments:
- "Nobody really cares what I think."
- "I need somebody to listen to my ideas rather than just tell me what to do."
- "I don't have all the answers. Can I help my friend anyway?"

SESSION GOALS

You'll help each group member
1. discover how hard it is to listen well,
2. examine the destructive effects of too much talk and the constructive results of good listening,
3. practice using listening skills.

SPECIAL PREPARATION

_____ Bring extra Bibles, small and large paper, markers, masking tape, and pencils.
_____ Arrange chairs in rows of six.
_____ Have in mind at least one youth who would be a confident storyteller for "Lousy Listener." Decide whether to contact this person ahead of time.
_____ Duplicate Workout Sheets #9 and #10.
_____ Bring masking tape and labels for "Listening with All of You."
_____ Sample situations for "Listening Practice."

BUILDING THE BODY

Try one of these activities to build group members' listening skills.

FUZZY CONNECTION

Seat group members in chairs which are arranged in rows of about six. Say: **I will whisper a message to the first person in each row and that person will whisper it to the next in line until the one at the end receives the message. This last person will write the message word for word as received. Listen carefully so the message will be passed accurately!** Emphasize that they cannot repeat the message or ask questions. Whisper Ephesians 4:29 to the first youth: "Do not let any unwholesome talk come out of your mouths, but only what is helpful for building others up according to their needs, that it may benefit those who listen." Then take paper and pencils to the ends of the rows and remind the final listeners to write the message word for word as they received it.

When the message has been passed, call for the final listeners to read what they received. Encourage everyone to compare those messages with what they received and passed. After several have shared, explain that the message was Ephesians 4:29. Ask: **Why were there differences? What would have helped you hear and understand what the person before you really said?** Write their ideas on a chalkboard or large piece of paper. Supplement with these tips: **The message would have been better understood if we could have asked questions, repeated what the other said to be sure we understood, and passed the message in short sections instead of such a long verse.**

Explain: **Listening is more than closing your mouth. It is a two-way process of understanding. In this session we'll discover and practice several elements of listening. We'll find out why listening is one of the best ways to help a friend with a problem. In the next three sessions we'll focus on other helping skills, giving advice, and where to find more help.**

LISTEN TO LEARN

Direct youth to close their eyes and, if your space is adequate, to sit or lie on the floor. Instruct them: **For the next 60 seconds, listen for as many sounds as you can hear.** When a minute has passed ask them to tell you everything they heard. Then ask: **What did each of these sounds tell you?** (Examples: the children laughing told me they were enjoying their study; the car brakes told me an accident almost occurred.)

Explain: **Listening can teach not only you, but also the friend to whom you are listening. As your friend tells you his ideas and feelings, he understands them better. As you ask questions and then listen to your friend's answers, he feels motivated to do the right thing. Today we'll discover why listening is one of the best ways to help a friend with a problem. In the next three sessions we'll focus on other helping skills, on giving advice, and on where to find more help.**

LAUNCHING THE LESSON

PROBLEM ALPHABET

Group youth into teams of four to six and give them large sheets of paper and markers. You may want to divide the teams by birthdays: all the January, February, and March birthdays on one team, and so on. Direct the teams: **Write the alphabet vertically on the paper. Beginning with each letter of the alphabet, write a problem young people have. Spelling doesn't count and you can use words that sound like the letter as well as that actually begin with it. Examples include: Alcoholism, Boredom, Can't find a date, Divorce . . . Xpectations of parents are too high.**

Call for youth to hang their posters on the wall with masking tape. Explain: **During this four-week study we're going to focus on how we can help each other solve these problems.** (Keep the posters up throughout this study to give the group ideas for problems to address.)

Call on someone to read Philippians 4:13: "I can do everything through Him who gives me strength." Ask: **Whose power do we have for handling problems?** (Jesus' power.) Explain: **Jesus has not only the power, but He has the answers. The best problem-solving focuses on finding Jesus' answers. Listening is one way to help your friend do this.**

LOUSY LISTENER

Pull two empty chairs from the group, sit in one, and ask: **Who has a problem or something really exciting to tell? I'd like you to come sit in this chair right now and tell me about it.** (Choose someone with enough confidence to handle the following treatment. You may want to let her know ahead of time how you will treat her.)

When the person begins to talk, listen as poorly as possible. Demonstrate listening no-no's, such as: avoiding eye contact, turning away from the person, yawning, looking at your watch, fooling with your fingernails, doodling, interrupting to tell your story, failing to respond (for example, when she says she just got an A on a test, say, "What? I didn't hear you'), devaluing ("An A? That's nothing, I got one of those yesterday myself"), and more. Finally interrupt to say, "I'm sorry, I've got a class to teach," and stand up.

Direct all youth to open their Bibles to Romans 12:15: "Rejoice with those who rejoice; mourn with those who mourn." Call on a volunteer to read it aloud. Ask: **How well did I just practice this verse?** Encourage them to point out specific faults in your listening. **As they respond, write answers on the chalkboard.** After several flaws have been suggested, distribute Workout Sheet #9 to identify more listening blunders.

WORKOUT SHEET

Direct your group to separate the "Imitation Listening" principles from the

"Loving Listening" principles on Workout Sheet #9. They may want to work in pairs.

Review the "Loving Listening" principles (smile; respond; understand; pay attention; ask questions; nod in agreement; look into her eyes; turn toward the person; use interest words like "Really?" and "Oh!"; use prompters like "Then what?" and "What do you think?"; take the problem seriously, even if it would not bother you; repeat what your friend says in different words to be sure you understand) by asking: **How could I have demonstrated each of the principles of loving listening?** Clarify any unclear principles, such as: Interest words and prompters are words you use to encourage your friend to talk: "Uh-huh," "Then what?" "Really?" and more. **What other interest words and prompters do you use?** Direct youth to jot on their sheets examples of prompters and interest words that they use. (They will probably suggest current slang as well as "You're kidding.")

LOVING LISTENER

Challenge youth: **Who can listen better than I did? I invite you to listen to _______ as she retells her story. Practice the listening principles on Workout Sheet #9.**

After a youth accepts the challenge and listens, say: **How well did he listen? What positive listening principles did you notice? What could he have done to listen even better? Romans 12:15 advises us to "rejoice with those who rejoice" and "mourn with those who mourn." How does listening help us do this?** (Listening shows concern and empathy.)

Ask the storyteller: **Which person made you feel that you and your news were important? To which person would you go for help with a problem?** (The person who listened lovingly.)

STUDENT BOOK OPTION

Ask: **How does listening show love? Why is it often better to listen than to talk?** If you have the student book, direct youth to suggest how listening would minister to Greg, Diana, and Julia. Now turn your attention back to Workout Sheet #9. Write the names Greg, Diana, and Julia and underneath them, three loving listening actions that would help them solve their problems.

If you do not have the student book, call for volunteers to suggest several situations in which they like to be listened to and why.

EXPLORING THE WORD

Challenge youth to find a command about listening in James 1:19: "Everyone should be quick to listen, slow to speak and slow to become angry." Ask: **Why do you think James included this command?** (Because we talk too much; you can't take back your words once they're spoken; it takes lots of listening to understand what someone means.)

Say: **Could it be that we tend to talk too much and talk before we really understand? A man named Job had friends with that problem. Eager to help, they explained why they thought Job was having so many problems. Poor Job had lost his family, livestock, crops, and health. He suffered horribly. Though his friends meant well, they caused more problems than they solved. In fact, they made Job's pain worse. Let's search Job 13:1-16 and 16:1-5 for what Job WANTED from his friends and what he GOT.**

WORKOUT SHEET

Distribute Workout Sheet #10. Students should look up the verses given and write what Job wanted and got from his friends. Answers:

Job wanted:
- to be respected as an equal (13:2)
- to talk with God rather than be told how God feels (13:3)
- listening (13:5-6)
- his friends to listen to God (13:9-11)
- opportunity to talk and silent friendship (13:13)
- to trust God and talk with Him about his problems (13:15)
- his friends to believe that he was close to God (13:16)
- comfort (16:2)
- sympathy/empathy (16:4)
- comforting words (16:5)

Job got:
- lies from his friends (13:4)
- worthless advice (13:4; 13:12)
- inaccurate or confused understanding of God (13:7-8)
- misery rather than comfort (16:2)
- long-winded speeches (16:3)
- critical head-shaking (16:4)

Reread Job 13:15. Point out Job's absolute confidence in God. Job fussed and complained a lot, but his trust in God never failed. Point out 13:5-7, which states that his friends did not understand as well as they thought they did. Emphasize: **One of the dangers of talking is that we might not fully understand the situation. Misunderstanding could cause us to give wrong or dangerous advice. For example, if a friend's sweetheart broke off the relationship after a year, we might encourage the friend to try to get back together. In truth the breakup opens the way for the person God wants for your friend. Your listening can encourage your friend to discover and follow God's will.**

Encourage your group to read the entire Book of Job this week for details about Job's struggle with problems. Explain that Satan was the source of his trouble, and encourage them to notice ways Job responded to his troubles.

LISTENING SHOWS LOVE

For each team of four to six people, post a large piece of paper with LISTEN written vertically. Direct them to complete the acrostic by writing a word or phrase beginning with each letter that tells how listening shows love. For example:

Listening can help a friend learn to solve his/her own problem
Imitates Jesus
Shows love
Tells that you care
Encourages your friend who
Needs a listening ear

APPLYING THE TRUTH

LISTEN WITH ALL OF YOU

If you have the student book, direct your youth to look at the listener on page 41. If you do not have the student book, call on a confident, fun-loving youth to stand in the center of the circle. Say: **Realizing that we use all of our bodies to listen, label ____ (name of youth) with listening instructions. Label at least his brain (head), eyes, eyebrows, mouth, shoulders, arms, hands, legs, and feet.** Examples include: On his hands tape, "Don't doodle while your friend is talking." On his feet tape, "Take a walk with your friend when he needs to talk." Youth may have ideas for labeling parts not discussed in this session. Provide paper and masking tape.

LISTENING PRACTICE

Divide youth into trios. Declare the one with the birthday closest to today the LISTENER. Declare the one with the birthday furthest from today the TALKER, and the other person the OBSERVER. Give these instructions: **TALKERS, tell about a problem you are currently facing, or use one of the sample situations I have in my hand.** (Have samples ready.) **LISTENERS, listen with the skills we have just discovered. OBSERVERS, watch to see how well the LISTENERS listen.** (HINT: Because this is a sensitive exercise, avoid placing critical youth with shy youth. Encourage positiveness. Letting youth choose their own groups may be best because they tend to choose people with whom they feel comfortable.)

Give the TALKER 90 seconds to talk. Then call time and direct the OBSERVER to tell the TALKER and LISTENER what he observed. Call for groups to share their experiences. Then direct the groups to trade roles. The OBSERVER now becomes the LISTENER, the LISTENER becomes the TALKER, and the TALKER becomes the OBSERVER. Repeat the same process.

Repeat the same process once more so that all youth play each role. Call the groups into one large circle to share new discoveries. Ask: **What have you learned about listening? About talking? About helping your friends with problems?** Allow plenty of time to share.

Close by praying that God would guide us to listen His way.

WORKOUT SHEET # 9

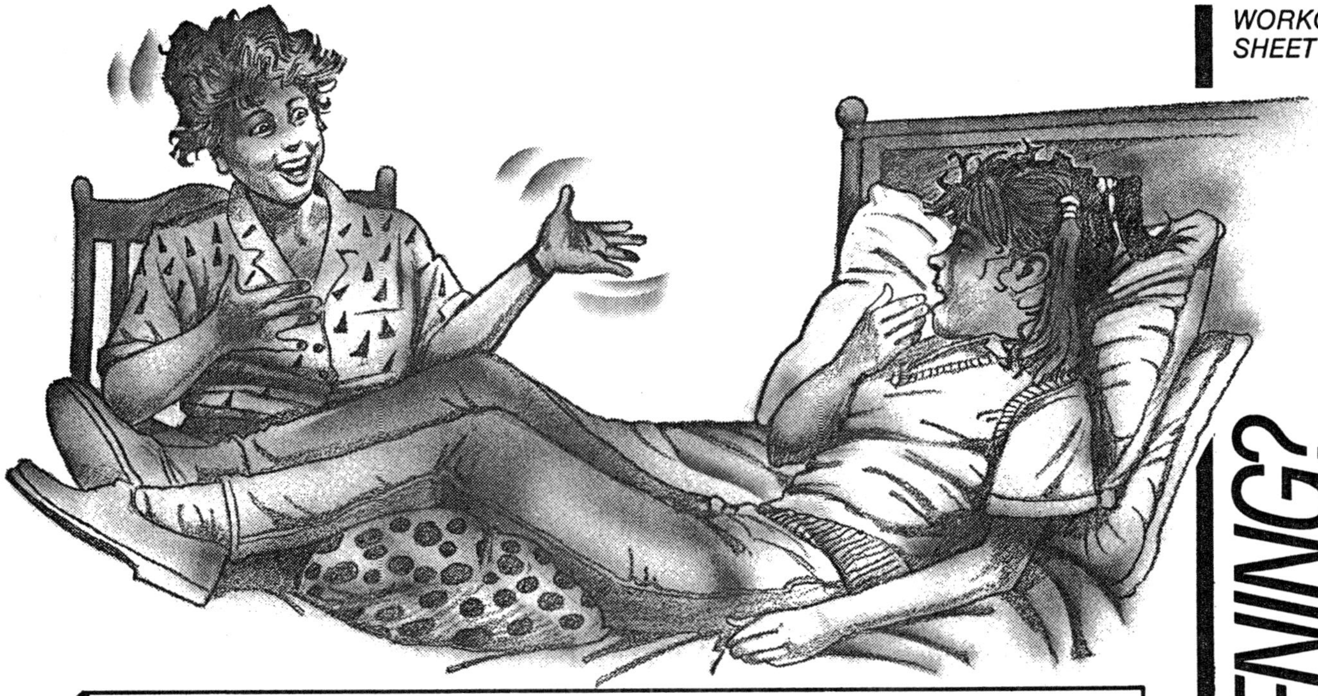

ARE YOU REALLY LISTENING?

CAN YOU TELL A FAKE FROM THE REAL THING?

Separate these listening behaviors into the categories "Imitation Listening" and "Loving Listening." Put a check in the appropriate column for each item. The imitation listener may close his mouth, but he certainly doesn't hear! The loving listener communicates God's love through active listening.

	IMITATION LISTENING	LOVING LISTENING
Pay attention		
Understand		
File your fingernails		
Look at your watch		
Think of what you'll say next		
Ask questions		
Respond		
Turn toward the person		
Turn away from the person		
Yawn		
Repeat what your friend says in different words		
Look into her eyes		
Explain away the problem		
Avoid eye contact		
Nod in agreement		
Use interest words ("Really?" "Oh!")		
Doodle		
Use prompters ("Then what?" "What do you think?")		
Smile		
Take the problem seriously, even if it would not bother you		
Interrupt to tell your story		

BE QUIET • A • N • D • LISTEN !

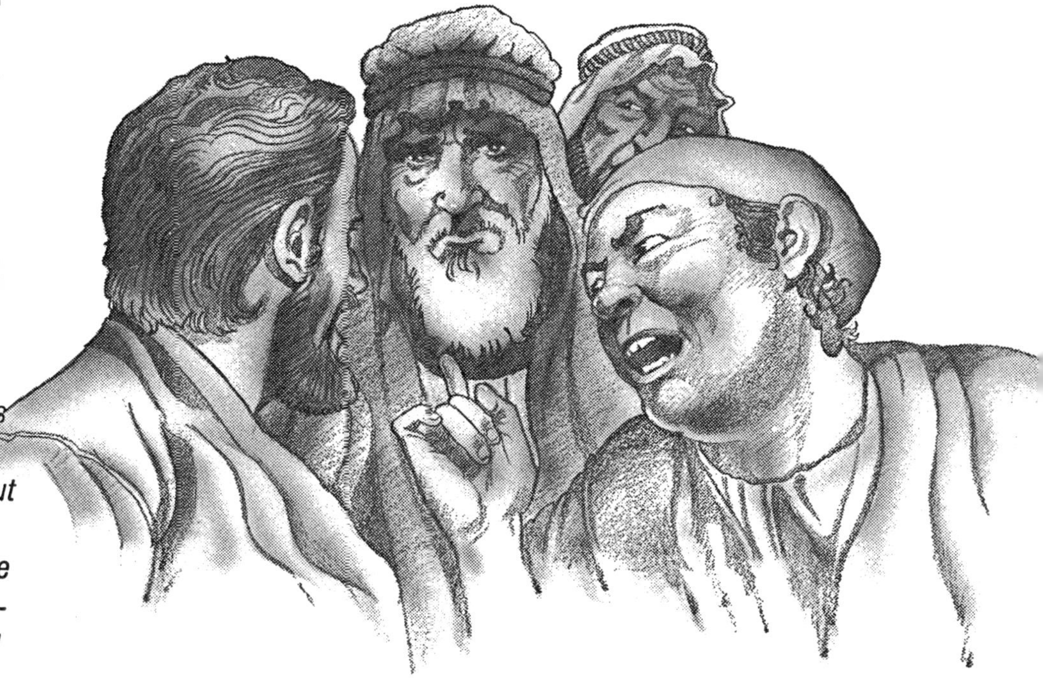

When Job was having more problems than we could ever imagine having, he wanted his friends to listen to him. But instead they talked too much—and said all the wrong things. Look up the verses from the Book of Job listed below and write what Job wanted *and what he* got.

JOB WANTED . . .

- 13:2 ______________________________
- 13:3 ______________________________
- 13:5-6 ______________________________
- 13:9-11 ______________________________
- 13:13 ______________________________
- 13:15 ______________________________
- 13:16 ______________________________
- 16:2 ______________________________
- 16:4 ______________________________
- 16:5 ______________________________

JOB GOT . . .

- 13:4 ______________________________
- 13:4, 12 ______________________________
- 13:7-8 ______________________________
- 16:2 ______________________________
- 16:3 ______________________________
- 16:4 ______________________________

SESSION 6

WORD POWER (Ephesians 4:29; selected passages)

KEY CONCEPT

Our words make our friends' problems better or worse. With conscious effort we can make that effect positive.

MEETING THE NEED

This session will respond to the following student comments:

- "I don't know what to say when my friends come to me with problems."
- "What I say doesn't make any difference anyway."
- "How did Jesus help with problems?"

SESSION GOALS

You will help each group member

1. recognize that words contribute to a friend's happiness or sadness,
2. examine ways Jesus helped,
3. practice using words to help rather than hurt.

SPECIAL PREPARATION

_____ Arrange chairs along the wall to allow room for a pyramid.
_____ Create the "Trading Game" by duplicating and cutting apart Workout Sheet #11.
_____ Write people-helping skills and corresponding passages on slips of paper, and post the three questions for "Learning from Jesus."
_____ Duplicate a copy of Workout Sheet #12 for each youth.
_____ Post the ABC listing of problems created in session 5.

BUILDING THE BODY

Open with one of these pyramid activities.

BUILD ME UP

Challenge groups of about 10 to build a human pyramid. Suggest this structure: Four get on hands and knees and kneel close together. Three get on hands and knees on top of this first level, placing one hand and one knee on one person and the other hand and knee on the person next to him. Two form a third level the same way. Finally, one kneels on the top of the pyramid. Youth may know of other pyramid forms which are equally effective. (NOTE: You can form a pyramid with as few as three people: two on the first level and one on the top level.)

When the pyramid is formed, ask: **What would happen if the top person started jumping? What if a bottom-level person decided to lie down? What if a second- or third-level person decided to tickle?** Pause at this point and call for youth to suggest other actions which might destroy the pyramid. (A sneeze, squirming, fatigue.) After they have suggested several, point out: **Even tiny actions make or break the pyramid. Some are intentional, like tickling, and some are accidental, like sneezing.** Then ask: **What actions make sure our pyramid stands strong and straight?** (Staying still, encouraging each other, balancing the load, concentrating on your part.)

Say: **Just as each person is important to the success or failure of this pyramid, each of you is important to your friend's happiness. Your words and actions will help her solve her problems, or make them worse. You can build her up or cut her down. You can help carry her load, or add to it. Just as in the pyramid, some destructive actions are unintentional: you might not mean to say your friend's problem is dumb—you're just in a bad mood. But it hurts your friend just the same. Let's be intentional about our friend-helping. You and your friends are depending on each other!**

LET'S BUILD TOGETHER

If your space is limited or your youth are not dressed for building a human pyramid, build your pyramid with blocks on a table. Give each person a block and instruct: **Using all your blocks, build a pyramid.** When the pyramid is formed, ask: **What would happen if someone pulled a bottom block out? What if, rather than contributing to the pyramid, someone threw his block at the completed pyramid? What if someone bumped the table?** Pause at this point and call for youth to suggest other actions which might destroy the pyramid. (Pyramid not balanced; one block accidentally out of place.) After youth have suggested several, point out: **Some of the actions we have suggested are intentional, like pulling a block, and some are accidental, like bumping the table. Even a tiny bump could disrupt the pyramid.** Then ask: **What actions make sure our pyramid stands strong and straight?** (Working together to make it steady, balancing the load, contributing your block.) Make the remarks in the closing paragraph under "Build Me Up."

LAUNCHING THE LESSON

IT HAPPENS EVERY DAY

Pull the chairs into a circle. Make each statement given below and direct youth to stand after each that is true:

1. You talked about a problem today.
2. You listened to a problem today.
3. You asked for help with a problem during the past week.
4. You solved a problem today.
5. You have no problems today.

Explain: **Problems are a daily part of life, and solving them right takes a lot of skill and understanding. We can stand with our friends to help them solve their problems.**

TRADING GAME

Before the session, duplicate four copies of Workout Sheet #11, cut the copies on the lines, and shuffle them. This creates a matching game for 12 youth. If you have more than 12 group members, duplicate more copies. If you have less than 12, choose the helping skills you feel are most important. You need four matching cards per person.

The game guides youth to memorize helping skills. Give each person four different cards. Explain: **In your hands are four cards. On each is a helping action and a definition. The cards in your hand do not now match. When I say "go," obtain a set of four matching cards by trading one card at a time. As you trade, do not tell what is on the card. The first one to complete a set yells the name of the helping action on the card. Any questions?** Pause for questions. Then say, "Go!" When the first match is made, encourage youth to continue to trade until all actions are yelled.

Ask: **Who can name all 12 helping skills?** Encourage several volunteers to try. Clarify skills that might be unfamiliar using the brief definitions on the cards. Point out: **Because you have been involved in trading and looking at the cards repeatedly, you remember. In a similar way, spending time with your friends helps you remember what helps them. You can help a friend using helping actions, such as giving advice, listening, or both. Working together, you can find the helping actions that solve the problem best.**

EXPLORING THE WORD

LEARNING FROM JESUS

To help group members discover some of Jesus' people-helping skills, say: **How did Jesus respond when people came to Him with problems? In**

a moment, I'll give you a passage telling about a time Jesus helped someone with a problem. He used each of the 12 skills we learned in the trading game. (In fact, the Bible was the source of these helping actions!) As you read your passage find the skills Jesus used. Answer the three posted questions and then, concentrating on the suggested skill, prepare to present a brief skit demonstrating that helping skill Jesus used. You may use the Scripture passage as your skit script (question 1) or create a skit showing how you would use the skill today (question 3). (NOTE: You may want to give the longer passages to youth who are more comfortable with reading.)

Distribute these passages to teams of at least two. (If you have less than 24 youth, select the passages you feel are most important.)

A. SHOW ACCEPTANCE: John 4:4-26
B. ASK QUESTIONS: Matthew 16:13-20
C. LISTEN: Matthew 3:13-15
D. RESPOND TO FEELINGS: John 6:16-21
E. REJECT THE SIN BUT NOT THE PERSON: John 8:2-11
F. EMPATHIZE: John 11:1-3, 17-44
G. UNDERSTAND: John 15:18-26
H. FIND THE REASON FOR THE PROBLEM: John 16:17-31
I. SUGGEST AND EVALUATE POSSIBLE SOLUTIONS: John 6:5-13
J. ENCOURAGE: John 21:15-19
K. STAND BY YOUR FRIEND: John 12:1-8
L. COMFORT: John 14:1-7

Post these questions:
1. What words and actions did Jesus use to show this helping skill?
2. What other helping skills did Jesus demonstrate? (not limited to the 12 we learned in the matching challenge)
3. Name a similar situation youth face and words or actions you would use to demonstrate this same helping skill in that situation.

Call for each team to answer the three questions and then present its skit. Sample answers:

SHOW ACCEPTANCE: John 4:4-26—(1) "Will you give me a drink?" He asked for water from the woman even though others disapproved of her (v. 27). (2) Asked questions, answered questions, used regular conversation to lead to spiritual things, rejected the sin but not the person. (3) Racial prejudice or cliques at school. I could make friends with someone others reject by talking with the person.

ASK QUESTIONS: Matthew 16:13-20—(1) "Who do people say the Son of Man is?" and "Who do you say I am?" (2) Praised Peter for a wise answer. Told him the good that would come from believing and understanding Jesus. (3) My friend can't decide what to do. I could ask my friend, "What have other people said you should do?" "What do you think you should do?" "What do you think Jesus wants you to do?"

LISTEN: Matthew 3:13-15—(1) He listened to John to understand both his words and his feelings. (2) He answered his questions directly. He encouraged him to obey God in this matter. (3) My friend is worried about what will happen if she does the right thing. I could listen to her fears, reassure her, and then encourage her to do right.

RESPOND TO FEELINGS: John 6:16-21—(1) "It is I; don't be afraid." Calmed fears by assuring them that He was with them. (2) Refused to criticize them for feeling afraid; didn't accuse them of having no faith. (3) My friend is really sad about her boyfriend breaking up with her. I can be with her and let her cry when she needs to.

REJECT THE SIN BUT NOT THE PERSON: John 8:2-11—(1) He kept silent for awhile after she was accused and then said, "If anyone of you is without sin, let him be the first to throw a stone at her." (2) Did not condemn her; told her to stop sinning. (3) My friend is sleeping with his girlfriend and he talks to me about it. I could gently explain that sex before marriage causes more problems than it solves and that God wants him to wait until marriage. I could assure him of my friendship no matter what he does.

EMPATHIZE: John 11:1-3, 17-44—(1) "Your brother will rise again." "I am the resurrection and the life. He who believes in Me will live, even though he dies; and whoever lives and believes in Me will never die." (2) Cried along with Martha and Mary; listened; reassured them (v. 25); called for belief (vv. 25, 40). (3) My friend's grandfather died. I can go to her house and spend time with her. I can listen. I can assure her of everlasting life for believers.

UNDERSTAND: John 15:18-26—(1) Explained reason for the disciples' problem: "If the world hates you, keep in mind that it hated Me first. . . . I have chosen you out of the world. . . . They hated Me without reason." (2) Sympathized, understood, felt along with. (3) My friend is being treated unfairly. I can understand her feelings and help her find the reason for the unfair treatment: maybe the abuser is taking his unhappiness out on my friend.

FIND THE REASON FOR THE PROBLEM: John 16:17-31—(1) "Are you asking one another what I meant when I said . . . ? I tell you the truth, you will weep and mourn while the world rejoices. . . . I have told you these things, so that in Me you may have peace. In this world you will have trouble. But take heart! I have overcome the world" (vv. 19-20, 33). (2) Explained the truth using illustrations; didn't falsely reassure; was honest even though the truth was hard. (3) My friend's parents are divorcing. I can say, "It will be hard, but joy will come again someday. God will always be with you."

SUGGEST AND EVALUATE POSSIBLE SOLUTIONS: John 6:5-13—(1) Asked Philip, "Where shall we buy bread for these people to eat?" (2) Involved Philip in the solution: gathering up the food after people had eaten. (3) My friend is facing a huge problem. We could list possible solutions and pray for God's will (which might include a miracle!).

ENCOURAGE: John 21:15-19—(1) Asked, "Do you truly love Me?" and then told him what to do to demonstrate that love: "Feed My lambs." (2) Kept loving Peter even though Peter had denied Him three times; asked questions to teach him a point; used words that were important to their friendship: "Follow Me" was the same phrase Jesus used when He first invited Peter to be His disciple (Mark 1:17). (3) My friend has hurt me or someone I love. I can understand why it happened, forgive him, and restore our relationship.

STAND BY YOUR FRIEND: John 12:1-8—(1) When someone accused Mary of waste, Jesus understood and said, "Leave her alone. It was meant that she should save this perfume for the day of My burial." (2) Understanding; compliments. (3) Someone falsely accuses my friend or spreads a rumor. I can stand up for him and spread the truth rather than the rumor.

COMFORT: John 14:1-7—(1) Comforted them with true words, "I am going there to prepare a place for you." (2) Listened to His disciples' worries (chapter 13); answered their questions. (3) When a friend is upset about a Christian family member dying, I can assure him that God will take care of the person in heaven.

APPLYING THE TRUTH

WATCH YOUR WORDS

Point out: **We cannot overestimate the value of words in helping. Sometimes we use them too much, sometimes too little. But whenever we use them, let's be sure they help solve the problem rather than add to it. Ephesians 4:29-32 lists some ways we can use words. What are they?** (Build others up according to their needs; benefit those who listen; grieve the Holy Spirit of God; create bitterness, rage, anger, brawling [fighting], slander [defaming someone through criticism, rumors, or false talk], malice; create kindness, compassion, forgiveness.) **Which of these would help problems? Which would make them worse?**

WORKOUT SHEET

Distribute Workout Sheet #12, "Watch Your Words!" Instruct youth: **Circle "make it worse" words you tend to use. Add others you use that aren't on this list.** Give them a minute or two to do so. Emphasize that they will have to share their answers.

Next, instruct youth: **Draw a line from the "make it worse" words to "problem-solving" words that could replace them.** Call for volunteers to share examples of problem-solving words that could replace specific "make it worse" words.

To encourage youth, direct them: **Put a star by some helpful words you already use.** After a minute or two, say: **You already do some things well. Now improve on them!**

STUDENT BOOK OPTION

Say: **Let's apply what we've learned to some actual problems. On pages 48-49 of your student book are some sample problems. Write a letter to one of these people using the helpful actions we matched earlier and the "problem-solving" words on Workout Sheet #12.**

If you do not have the student book, let youth write about one of the problems on last week's ABC problem list or anonymously write one of their own problems.

Call for group members to read their problems and response letters. Point out one or more helping actions each person has used in his letter. Pray, thanking God for guiding us in our friend-helping.

TRADING GAME

Duplicate one copy of this sheet for every three group members. Cut the copies on the lines, creating cards to be used in the trading game.

SHOW ACCEPTANCE We feel more confident to solve problems when we're accepted.	**ASK QUESTIONS** They help you understand the problem and give your friend ideas for solutions.
LISTEN Your friend knows the problem better than you do.	**RESPOND TO FEELINGS** They're as important as words! Let your friend be comfortable crying and showing other emotions with you.
REJECT THE SIN BUT NOT THE PERSON Don't ignore wrong, but assure your friend of your love.	**EMPATHIZE** See things from your friend's point of view. Feel with your friend.
UNDERSTAND Listen and restate what you hear until you understand. Let your friend know you understand.	**FIND THE REASON FOR THE PROBLEM** When you know the source it's easier to attack and solve the problem.
SUGGEST AND EVALUATE POSSIBLE SOLUTIONS List lots of ideas and anticipate the probable results of each.	**ENCOURAGE** You give your friend confidence to solve the problem when you express your confidence in her.
STAND BY YOUR FRIEND Even when you don't know just what to do, your consistent friendship will help in many ways.	**COMFORT** Use true words ("God will take care of you no matter what happens") rather than false assurance ("He'll get better") to comfort your friend. Hugs are nice too!

WATCH *your* WORDS!

Every word you say has power. Your words can create or destroy, encourage or discourage, help or hurt. Circle "make it worse" words you tend to use. Notice the "problem-solving" words you could use to replace them, and put a star by some helpful words you already use. Commit yourself to using them even more effectively.

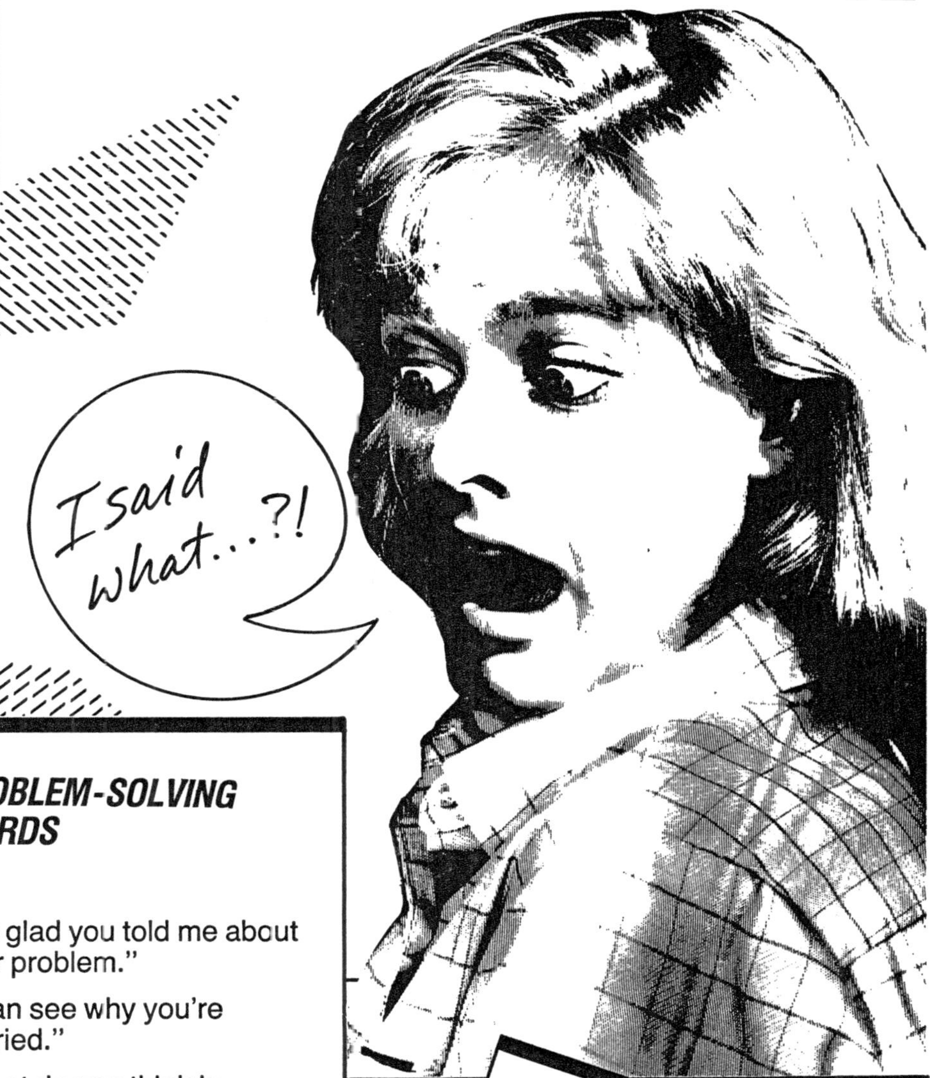

"MAKE IT WORSE" WORDS	***PROBLEM-SOLVING WORDS***
"I don't see why you're worried about that!"	"I'm glad you told me about your problem."
"That's no big deal."	"I can see why you're worried."
"Do this."	"What do you think is best?"
"You'd better not do that."	"What do you think will happen if you try that?"
"How did you get yourself into this mess?"	"What do you think caused the problem?"
"I can't believe you did that!"	"I'm concerned about you."
"What you did was wrong."	"It was wrong, but I still love you."
"Grow up!"	"How can I help you?"
"You'd better change before it gets worse!"	"Let's see if we can find the reason you're involved in this."
"A Christian wouldn't act that way!"	"What do you think Jesus wants you to do?"
"God is upset with you!"	"I know God wants to help you."

"Do not use harmful words, but only helpful words, the kind that build up and provide what is needed, so that what you say will do good to those who hear you."

Ephesians 4:29

WHAT'S YOUR PROBLEM?

SESSION 7

ADVICE IS NICE (SOMETIMES) (Selected passages)

KEY CONCEPT

Good advice results from understanding the problem and being in touch with the Advice-giver.

MEETING THE NEED

This session will respond to the following student concerns:
- "My friend asked me for advice. What do I say?"
- "Why does some advice bug me?"
- "Everyone has a different opinion. Which one is right?"

SESSION GOALS

You'll help each group member
1. discover pros and cons of giving advice,
2. match tips about giving advice to the Bible verses which explain them,
3. practice giving advice through asking questions and through other tips discovered in the session.

SPECIAL PREPARATION

_____ Bring wrapped lamp shade with sock inside for "Things Aren't Always as They Seem."
_____ Bring envelope with PRO and CON slips, and a watch with a second hand.
_____ Duplicate Workout Sheets #13 and #14.
_____ Cut out tips and verses on separate cards for the "Tips from the Master" concentration game.
_____ Bring extra Bibles, paper for three steps, and pencils.
_____ Post the ABC listing of problems created in session 5.

BUILDING THE BODY

THINGS AREN'T ALWAYS AS THEY SEEM

In the center of the group, place a sock inside a lamp shade wrapped in paper. Write these four questions on the chalkboard:

1. What is it?
2. What is it doing here?
3. Where should it be?
4. Who is the best person to put it there?

Distribute paper and direct youth to jot down their answers to the questions on the chalkboard. After a minute or two, ask the questions and call for answers. Encourage any who disagree with the majority to say so. Unwrap the shade and pull out the sock that is taped inside it. Explain that the sock is what you had in mind when you asked the questions. Give a brief summary of the answers, such as: **The sock got lost during the last outing and it is here to find its owner. It should be in the drawer of its owner, and the best person to put it there is the one who lost it.**

Amid youth protests of "Not fair!" explain: **Things are not always as they seem. The answers to these questions seemed obvious by the shape of the package. But we had to open the wrappings and dig deeper to find the true answers. The person who can best explain this sock is the person who lost it! How does this relate to giving advice to friends with problems?** Supplement youth ideas with these:

- Looking beneath the surface can give you information needed to solve problems successfully.
- We may think we know the answer to a problem, but we may be wrong.
- Until we ask questions, we won't always know how to help a friend solve a problem.
- After listening you'll better understand the problem.
- Your friend probably knows the most details about the problem.
- The best advice involves both you and your friend in finding a solution.

LAUNCHING THE LESSON

DEBATE

Post this statement: ADVICE HELPS MORE THAN IT HURTS.

Say: **When is giving advice a good idea? When is it dangerous? Let's debate the pros and cons of giving advice. Notice the two tables I have set up. One is labeled PRO and one is labeled CON. On each table are Bibles and paper on which to record your ideas. I have suggestions for both sides to start you thinking. Draw a slip of paper from this envelope to determine the side you will take. There is an equal number of PRO and CON slips in the envelope. No matter how you feel about advice-giving, try to come up with the most evidence for your side. If you are PRO, prove why advice helps more than it**

hurts. If you are CON, prove the opposite: that advice hurts more than it helps. I'll be available to help. There will be 3 minutes to prepare for the debate, 90 seconds to present your evidence, 1 minute to prepare for rebuttal, and 45 seconds for rebuttal. Any questions? After questions, direct youth to draw a slip and prepare for the debate. Go back and forth between tables, spending an equal amount of time at each. Encourage youth to think of their own ideas by giving hints (see suggestions below). Encourage teams to choose one main speaker but to plan to add ideas as he talks.

Proceed with the debate according to the instructions. Encourage them as they speak by interjecting, "Good point!" and similar comments every now and then. When one side feels tempted to argue, encourage them to write that point down for their rebuttal. Lend your assistance, but be sure youth talk more than you do.

After the debate, ask: **Who won this debate?** Let youth argue a bit over who was right. Point out: **This is an excellent debate topic because there is so much evidence on both sides.** Review the pros and cons of giving advice, including these suggestions:

PRO
1. Your advice may be right.
2. When your friend doesn't know what to do, your advice can give ideas for action.
3. Good advice can help your friend solve his own problem.
4. God's advice works for everyone. If we hear His advice right, our advice will be right. Be sure all advice agrees with the Bible.
5. Good advice can encourage your friend to live God's way.

CON
1. Your advice may be wrong.
2. What worked for you may not work for your friend.
3. Your friend may depend on you to solve his problems rather than doing it alone. (You want him to depend on God, not on you.)
4. God's advice always works, but we might misunderstand and give advice God would not give.
5. Your friend may blame you if the advice causes problems.

WORKOUT SHEET

Distribute Workout Sheet #13, "Dealing Out Advice." Explain: **Many factors affect whether to give advice or not. We'll illustrate this with a deck of factor cards. Some of the factors are contributed by the advice-giver, as you see in the first set of cards. Others are contributed by the advice-receiver, as in the second set. Put together the six factors that most characterize the last advice you received and write them on the blank hand of cards.** Encourage youth to combine their own attitudes and feelings and the actions and attitudes of the friend who gave advice. After youth have completed their hands, call on volunteers to share answers to these questions:

- **What six factors made up your "hand"?**
- **How did you feel about the advice? How did the factors create that feeling?** (For example, a know-it-all attitude made you angry.)

- **Was it good advice? What factors made it good?** (For example, it was good because my friend listened to my ideas as well as sharing his.)
- **What six factors do you think would make the strongest hand?**

Supplement responses to the last question with these factors:

1. **The advice agrees with the Bible.**
2. **The receiver wants advice.**
3. **The advice-giver demonstrates a loving attitude.**
4. **The advice-giver understands the problem well.**
5. **The receiver checks advice with the Bible before following it.**
6. **The receiver wants to solve the problem.**

EXPLORING THE WORD

TIPS FROM THE MASTER

Write the verses and tips from page 53 on separate cards, or duplicate the page and cut the cards out. Shuffle them and lay them out face down like a concentration game. Youth take turns turning over two cards to make a match. Because they will have to read the verses from their Bibles to see if the cards match, this activity is good Bible study. If your group is large you'll want to make more than one concentration game. The verses are listed beside their matches.

Display the concentration game and direct youth: **Each of these cards has a Bible passage or a tip about giving advice. Find out what the Bible says about giving advice by taking turns turning over two cards to make a match. If you match correctly, keep the cards. If not, turn them back over. Keep your Bible open to read the verses and verify the matches. Notice that the tips paraphrase what the verses tell us about advice.**

Provide opportunity to share examples of using the tips by asking: **Can you think of a situation in which you used one of these Bible verses or tips?** Push no one to answer and encourage the whole group to share examples on any tip. Discourage youth from giving names or telling details that would turn sharing into gossiping.

NOTE: Leave the matches correctly displayed for the application portion of this session.

OPTION: Point out: **Some people wanted Jesus' help and others didn't. The Matthew 22:15 tip reminds us that the Pharisees did not want Jesus' wisdom. You may have a friend you are concerned about who does not seem to want your help. How might you help that friend the way Jesus helped those who didn't want His help?** Supplement responses by explaining that when Jesus worked with Pharisees and others who misunderstood Him, He asked probing questions and encouraged them to think about their actions and beliefs. Though it is easier to help a friend who wants your help, you can offer help to those who don't want it. Just keep in mind that they may misunderstand you. Ask: **What questions might you ask to gently encourage your friend to think about her actions and give her courage to do the right thing?**

Proverbs 27:9	People like to hear the advice of their friends.	Proverbs 11:14	You'll more likely make the right choice when you get lots of advice.
Proverbs 10:11-14	Choose carefully who you get advice from. Some people's words will do you good; others' will harm you.	Proverbs 12:15	A fool listens only to his own advice.
Ecclesiastes 10:14	No human knows the future. (Therefore we can ultimately trust only God, not human advice.)	Psalm 19:12-14	Friends can help each other see mistakes they don't see in themselves.
Nehemiah 8:8	The best advice helps people understand what God expects.	2 Chronicles 10:6-7, 13-14, 18	Often people with more experience give better advice.
Hebrews 10:24	The best advice encourages love and living God's way.	Matthew 22:15	Words can be twisted. Repeat what you think they mean to be sure of the message.

LET'S FIND MORE

Explain: **The verses we've just studied are just a few of the many verses on how to give and seek good advice. I'll give you five minutes to search the Book of Proverbs for more. Write the verse reference and a quick note about what it says. Choose a partner or two to work with. The team with the longest list wins.** Provide paper, extra Bibles, pencils, and encouragement. Suggest that youth keep an eye out for such words as "wise," "wisdom," "counsel," "advice," "friend," and "fool."

Call for teams to share their findings by taking turns saying a verse and its contents. Encourage youth to jot down verses other teams found that were not on their own lists.

APPLYING THE TRUTH

STUDENT BOOK OPTION

Explain: **One of the best ways to give advice is to guide your friend to discover God's answer for herself. You can do this through asking questions.**

If your group is using the student book, direct them to circle all the questions used by Sheila on pages 50-51. Ask: **How did these questions help Elise solve her problem?**

WORKOUT SHEET

Rather than or in addition to the student book option, distribute Workout Sheet #14 and direct youth: **In the space provided, write a problem you or a friend face. You might want to choose a problem from the ABC listing we made in session 5. Don't sign your name—the problems will be anonymous. In a moment I'll collect and shuffle the papers and pass them out so that no one has his own paper.**

Collect the problems. Shuffle and redistribute them. Direct the new owners: **Write advice concerning the problem using the questions on the worksheet, the helpful actions we matched during our Bible study time (they are displayed where you matched them to jog your memory), and the good advice factor cards on Workout Sheet #13.**

Return the worksheets to their original owners. Call for volunteers to read their problems and advice.

Close by praying that Jesus, the best advice-giver, would guide our advice-giving and our friend-helping.

DEALING OUT ADVICE

WORKOUT SHEET # 13

Giving advice is not a simple "do or don't" dilemma. Instead you take into account all the factors in a situation to decide whether and how to give advice. Below the hand of blank cards on this sheet are decks of advice-giving and advice-receiving factor cards. Think about the last time someone gave you advice. Build your hand by writing in the six factors (cards) that were most influential in how you received that advice.

Advice disagrees with the Bible

Advice is right

Loving attitude

Understands the problem well

Has listened to the friend's ideas

Advice is wrong

DEALT BY THE ADVICE-GIVER:

Talks more than the friend

Advice agrees with the Bible

Feels his way is the only way

Know-it-all attitude

Encourages dependence on God, not self

DEALT BY THE ADVICE-RECEIVER:

Wants advice

Trusts the advice-giver

Does not trust the advice-giver

Prays and thinks over the advice before following it

Follows advice blindly

Refuses to make own decisions

Does not want to solve the problem

Blames advice-giver if things don't work out

Wants listening ear, not advice

Checks the advice against the Bible

Wants to solve the problem

WHAT'S THE QUESTION?

Asking questions is one of the most valuable ways of helping your friend solve a problem. Jot down a problem someone told you about recently and write at least three questions that could help your friend discover solutions to the problem. Possibilities are listed below.

- How do you feel about it?
- What do you want most to happen?
- What actions and attitudes could make that happen? How could you contribute to making it happen?
- Who is involved besides you? How do they affect your choices?
- What are your options?
- What have other people told you to do?
- What do you think is best?
- What will happen if you try that option? The other ones?
- What have you already tried? What were the results?
- What is the worst that could happen?
- What is the best that could happen?
- What does the Bible say about it?
- What do you think Jesus wants you to do?
- Why is obeying God worth the risk?

PROBLEM:

ADVICE:

SESSION 8

SERIOUS HELP FOR SERIOUS PROBLEMS (Mark 9:17-29)

KEY CONCEPT

The best friend-helpers recognize when problems are too big to solve alone and know where to find more help.

MEETING THE NEED

This session will respond to the following student concerns/comments:
- "My friend is in big trouble. How do I get her out of it?"
- "What do I do when I don't know how to help?"
- "Who can I trust when my friend needs more help than I can give?"

SESSION GOALS

You'll help each group member
1. overcome some common misconceptions about helping friends,
2. discover elements the disciples lacked and elements youth lack in their helping,
3. pinpoint specific ways to help with serious problems.

SPECIAL PREPARATION

_____ Arrange chairs in one large circle.
_____ Bring pitcher and paper sacks with contents (described under "All for One, One for All").
_____ Bring extra Bibles and pencils.
_____ Duplicate Workout Sheets #15 and #16.

BUILDING THE BODY

ALL FOR ONE, ONE FOR ALL

Prior to the session, arrange a table (or floor) with a paper sack at each place and a large empty pitcher in the center. The sacks should look alike, but the contents will be different. Divide these materials among the sacks: knives, peanut butter, jelly, bread, cups, lemonade mix, water for lemonade, sugar for lemonade, a spoon to stir the lemonade, napkins.

As youth arrive instruct them to take a seat but not look in the sacks. When all have been seated, explain: **I have provided a snack to begin our session. Please open your sacks and enjoy it!** Resist giving help. Let them discover how to share the materials so all have an equal snack.

After youth have worked together (or have refused to work together) to provide peanut butter and jelly sandwiches and lemonade, discuss the process by asking such questions as:

- **What was the object of this exercise?**
- **How did you know what to do?**
- **What were the results of working together?**
- **Who requested help? Who helped you?**
- **Did anyone refuse to cooperate? What happened then?**
- **Did anyone drink the water instead of contributing it to the lemonade? Did you notice that unless everyone poured the lemonade ingredients into the pitcher, it would not have tasted right?**

Ask: **What does this activity have to do with helping friends solve their problems?** Encourage youth to share their ideas. Supplement with:

- We can solve problems together we might not be able to solve alone.
- If you can't help, someone else probably can.
- Not everyone has the same type help to contribute.
- It may take several friends to help.
- Sometimes an extra helper can teach you what to do. Other times the extra helper must do the helping.

LAUNCHING THE LESSON

WHAT DO YOU THINK?

Direct youth to sit in one large circle. Explain: **I will read several statements. After I read a statement, stand if you think it is true. Stay seated if you think it is false. Try to trust your own understanding. The only one standing or sitting may be correct!** After each statement, encourage youth to share their reasons for standing or sitting. Briefly supplement their ideas by explaining why the statement is true or false.

1. **If a friend comes to me with a problem, I owe it to him to help him solve it myself.** (True and false: It is true that you want to help your friend, but that does not mean always doing the helping yourself. Calling on others to help is a way to help your friend.)

2. **People who threaten suicide really won't kill themselves.** (False: Talk about suicide is often serious. Listen and try to give hope: "You feel so sad today, but God has answers." Then tell an adult about the suicide threat. Ask what to do about it.)
3. **I betray my friend when I send him to someone else for help or ask advice for helping him.** (False: It often shows more love to get qualified help.)
4. **Drugs are not that big a problem anymore.** (False: In many areas drug usage is increasing and the drugs have more devastating effects.)
5. **If I ask an adult for help, he'll blab it to everyone.** (False: Many adults can be fully trusted. They respect you and want to help you help your friend. Many agencies offer confidential help.)
6. **A true Christian won't have any problem he and the Lord can't handle.** (True and false: It is true that God has all the answers, but because He often uses people to help us find those answers, it is false that a Christian never needs people to help.)
7. **When my friend has a really big problem, she'll probably tell me first.** (True: People go to their friends with problems before they approach professional counselors.)
8. **Youth don't have really big problems.** (False: Youth face depression, abuse, pregnancy, death, car accidents, imprisonment, suicide, tragedy, severe parent problems, and more.)
9. **A good friend can help a person get through really big problems.** (True: Even when your friend needs outside help, your friendship is one of the strongest factors in solving problems. Many major helping programs depend on the support and encouragement of peer groups.)

EXPLORING THE WORD

WHY THE PROBLEM?

Continue a similar learning method by reading Mark 9:17-29; youth should follow along. Instruct: **Keep your Bibles open to Mark 9:17-29. Stand when you find a verse that supports or disproves the statement I make.** Read these statements, one at a time, pausing briefly to discuss each. Suggested verses and comments are in parentheses.

- **Sometimes even the most well-intentioned friends (here the disciples) need more resources than their own.** (True, v. 18—The disciples could not heal the boy even though they had been able to heal others.)
- **Even though the father loved his son and wanted to help him, he could not heal him.** (True, vv. 17-18.)
- **Some people hinder God's work either intentionally or unintentionally.** (True, v. 19—The people failed to believe in Jesus; this somehow hindered the disciples' ability to heal.)
- **Jesus healed the boy immediately.** (Not true, vv. 20-21—Jesus talked with the father first, then cast out the spirit [vv. 25-26].)
- **Jesus was angry about the man's lack of faith.** (Not true, vv. 23-24—Rather than criticize the man's faith, Jesus encouraged him to look at his belief. The father trusted Jesus to increase his faith.)
- **The disciples asked Jesus why they couldn't drive out the spirit. Jesus said they weren't good enough friends.** (Not true, v. 29—Jesus said that kind of spirit could come out only through prayer. Because prayer is communication with God, apparently the disciples were de-

pending on their own power rather than God's power.)

- **Ultimately Jesus is the healer, no matter what person He works through.** (True, vv. 25-27, 29. Whether you, your friend, or a trusted adult solves the problem, the solution comes from Jesus.)

Ask: **What elements do we lack in our helping?** (Knowledge of how to handle difficult problems; not enough experience in solving big problems; no power over the people who are causing the problem, i.e., a friend's parent is being cruel and we cannot stop him; understanding the details of the problem, etc.) **What important element do we have for helping?** (Our friends trust us.) Explain: **One of the best ways to earn this trust is to learn to help and to find the best help possible.**

Call on two volunteers to read Proverbs 17:17 and Proverbs 18:24. Ask: **What do these verses assure us about friend-helping?** Supplement responses with: **Our love can encourage friends to find the strength they need to conquer problems (17:17), and we can stick by our friends in the midst of their problems (18:24).**

APPLYING THE TRUTH

WORKOUT SHEET

Explain that we give much of our help through talking: **As we studied in the second session, we become better friend-helpers when we choose the right words. When our friends encounter big problems, it is especially hard to know what to say. This Workout Sheet will give us practice choosing words that give our friends strength and show our friendship.** Distribute copies of Workout Sheet #15 and direct youth: **Circle the sentence in each trio that would most communicate love to your friends. Some will have more than one good possibility.** After a few minutes, call for volunteers to share their choice for each trio and why they chose it.

The best choices are probably:

A–3 (It is OK to question God because He always has an answer; humans don't become angels; we tread dangerously when we try to speak for God: "God did it because. . . . " Remember Job's friends!)

B–2 (If the person could "just quit" he wouldn't be hooked; he doesn't need accusations, he needs help.)

C (All three help the friend find solid answers but in addition to options 1 and 3, get adult help.)

D–2, 3 (Option 1 accuses, and accusations don't help.)

E (All are good responses but in addition, get adult help.)

F (All are good responses: 1 encourages gently; 2 assures that the problem won't be blabbed everywhere; 3 invites trust, but be cautious about promising confidentiality—you may have to tell your friend's name for his sake.)

After discussing the Workout Sheet, explain that our actions also communicate love. Ask: **What actions might accompany these words?** (Go with your friend to see the helper. Ask questions: "What did he say?" "How do you feel about it?" "What is the next step?" Tell your friend you are there to talk; spend time together; listen a lot.)

WHERE DO I FIND HELP?

To help youth learn how to help friends, present the following material in a minilecture, writing questions on the chalkboard as you talk:
When you're "shopping for a helper," you go about it like you would do other shopping. You search for quality, checking both the outer appearance and the unseen features:
- **Does he base his words and actions on the Bible?**
- **Does he seem competent?**
- **Will his advice hold up?**

You check to be sure the helper "fits" your needs and style:
- **Do you trust him?**
- **Do you like him?**
- **Do you feel comfortable with him?**
- **Does what he says make sense to you?**
- **Do you communicate well?**

You ask other people's opinions:
- **Has his advice worked for others?**
- **Has his advice caused problems for anyone else?**
- **Does he follow God?**

Of course it's always best to shop around and be on the lookout for good helpers before you need them. But if you're in a hurry, make the best purchase you can. Your minister or a Christian adult you've grown close to and trusted in the past are good candidates. Ask God to guide you in your choice.

Turn the discussion toward helping friends with grief. Ask questions and give new information to help present the material. Say: **Because we don't understand it, we tend to avoid helping our friends with grief. But by learning about and responding to grief, you can help your friend significantly, even without adult assistance. Any time we lose someone or something, we feel grief. What are some losses young people face that cause grief?** (Death of a friend or family member, moving, getting cut from the team, discovery of a serious disease, loss of a contest or position, breaking up with a boyfriend or girlfriend.)

The more important the person or position that is lost, the longer we grieve. Grieving can last up to a year. Signs of grief include shock, sadness, tears, feelings of loss, feeling worthless, feeling like nothing matters anymore, dreams that the loss has never occurred, and more. Only when we allow ourselves to have these sad feelings can we later truly feel happy again. Because feelings of grief are important healers, don't tell your friend to "get busy and stop thinking about it." Let him be sad and be sad with him. "Mourn with those who mourn" (Romans 12:15).

Here's a rhyme that helps us remember how to help friends through grief: CARE, SHARE, and BE THERE.

How can you show your friend you care? (You don't need to say anything profound or answer deep questions about why the loss occurred. Just say, "I care." Send cards. Say, "I'm sorry," or "I don't know what to say, but I want you to know I care." Actively express your love.)

How can you share yourself with your friend to help her through grief? (Share your time, ears, understanding, and similar experiences. Let your friend share with you her feelings, fears, hopes, needs.)

How can you "be there"? (Even if you feel uneasy about going to the funeral home when someone has died, go. If you don't know what to say when your friend's boyfriend dumps her, call anyway. When you stay away, your friend feels two losses—your friendship and the original loss.)

Care, share, and be there: these are three ways to help a friend going through grief. Notice that the tips don't include giving your friend pat answers or reasons why the loss occurred—that's not what people need. They just need to know you care that they hurt. Perhaps later they can explore good that has come out of grief and you can help them sort it out, but at first be careful to avoid brushing aside their pain by saying it's all for the best anyway.

WORKOUT SHEET

Distribute Workout Sheet #16, "Danger Signals." It is a handout that lists major problems youth face and signals which tell us a friend might have one of these problems. Go through the information on the sheet together and give examples and answer questions as needed.

Reinforce the material from the lecture/discussion and Workout Sheet #16 by asking these questions (students can draw answers from this session and from the student book): **Who is the first person your friend will come to for help?** (Me.) **Who can help you help your friend?** (Youth pastor, ministers, parents, Bible study teachers, Christian doctors, Christian counselors, school counselors, trusted adults.) **Who does a grieving friend need, and how can you help?** (He needs me—to care, share, and be there.) **Who do you trust who could help in time of need?** (Allow time for youth to think of an adult they would call on.)

For helping friends with specific problems, give group members these hot line numbers to write down on their Workout Sheets. For pregnancy, 1-800-BETHANY; for information about drugs, 1-800-241-7946 (gives ideas for drug-free fun, the effects of each drug, places to get help locally, how to discourage a friend from using drugs); for runaways, call a crisis line, National Runaway Switchboard, Trailways Bus Lines, a minister, etc.

Close this section of four studies by emphasizing: **The best way to help is to live according to the Bible, talk according to the Bible, listen the Bible's way, and give advice that guides your friend to follow the Bible. The only way you can do this is to be familiar with the Bible. I can't tell you "what we believe" and "what the Bible says" in these four brief sessions. You will have to study it for yourself. Read a chapter a day and pay attention at every Bible study you attend. Each time you read you'll understand better and will become a better friend-helper.** Thank youth for their contributions to the study and call for any final questions. Pray that God will help us to help others His way.

WHAT WOULD YOU SAY?

What do you say to a friend who needs help? Galatians 5:22-23 provides a marvelous guide for helping actions and attitudes. Translate these characteristics from the fruit of the Spirit into words by choosing the sentence in each trio that would be most helpful.

a Very upset about her mother's death, your friend says, "Why did God let this happen?" You say . . .
1. "You shouldn't question God!"
2. "He needed another angel."
3. "I don't know why God let it happen, but I do know that He feels your sadness along with you."

b Your friend confides, "I've been taking drugs and I'm afraid I'm hooked. I don't know what to do now." You say . . .
1. "Just quit. I know you can do it."
2. "Mr. Jessop said to call him if we ever needed help. Maybe he knows someone who can help us."
3. "I warned you not to get messed up in that stuff. Now look what has happened!"

c "I just can't stand it at home anymore. I know what my dad is doing to me is wrong, but there's nothing I can do to stop it. My only choice is to run away," says your friend. You say . . .
1. "What do you think might happen if you run away?"
2. "Let's try to find someone who can help you."
3. "Your feelings certainly make sense. I'd want to run too. But there's got to be a safer option."

d "I think I may be pregnant," worries your friend. You say . . .
1. "If you hadn't been sleeping with your boyfriend, this never would have happened."
2. "What makes you think you are pregnant?"
3. "Let's talk to my mom or your mom. They'll know what to do."

e "I think I'd be better off dead. At least then I'd be at peace and wouldn't have all these problems." You say . . .
1. "Right now all you feel is the pain of this world. If you kill yourself you'll also miss the joy. I know you don't believe it right now, but you will be able to solve this and happiness will return."
2. "The problems do seem overwhelming, don't they? What other choices do you see besides suicide?"
3. "I sure wouldn't be better off if you were dead! I'd miss you!"

f "When you suggest outside help, your friend resists, saying, "I came to you with this problem. I don't want anyone else to know!" You say . . .
1. "And I'm glad you did come to me. Because I want to help, I think we ought to try talking to ______. He understands us."
2. "There's a number you can call for confidential help."
3. "Would you mind if I talked to him without mentioning your name?"

"The fruit of the Spirit is love, joy, peace, patience, kindness, goodness, faithfulness, gentleness and self-control."

Galatians 5:22-23

DANGER SIGNALS

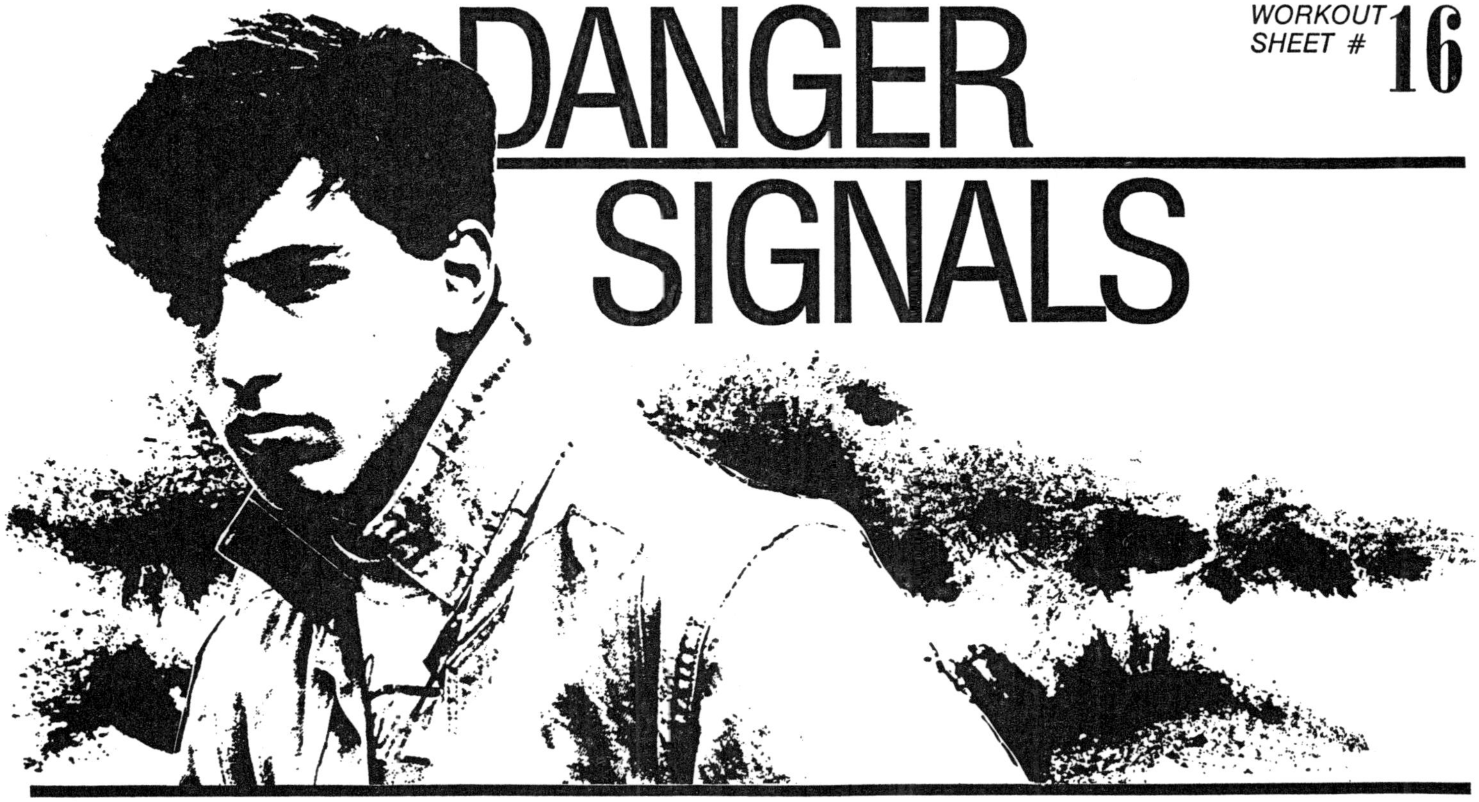

How do you know when a friend is having a serious problem? First, it helps to be aware of serious problems youth face, like these:

- Death of a loved one
- Depression
- Drug and alcohol abuse
- Sexual involvement
- Pregnancy
- Abuse
- Involvement in or victim of violence
- Suicidal feelings or attempts
- Severe parental or home problems

How will you know if your friend has one of these problems? Danger signals include:

- Not talking as much as before
- Change in friends
- Drop in grades
- Personality change
- Continuing depression
- Lowering or sudden extreme stiffening of moral standards
- Giving away prized possessions
- Extreme moodiness
- Sudden secretiveness or desire to be alone

When you notice one or more of these signals, what should you do? Take action:

- Let your friend know of your concern. "You seem upset lately. Do you want to talk?"
- Ask adult advice: "I'm worried about ____ because. . . . What should I do?"
- Actively accept your friend. When people feel loved and accepted by friends, they feel less need to seek acceptance through drugs, sex, or violence. Say, "Want to sit by me?" or "Come on—ride in our car!"
- Communicate your care through sending notes, by telephoning, or by talking in person. Say, "I care and God cares."
- Give hope: "God has answers. It may take a while, but we'll find them."

Think about your friends. ***Is someone sending these signals to you?***

WHAT'S OUR PROBLEM?

PART THREE

- Why does a good God allow evil?
- Why do bad things happen to good people?
- Why does God say no to everything fun?
- Why is the Christian life so hard?

These questions trouble most Christians at one time or another. Rather than being faith blockers, they can increase our confidence in God and draw us closer to Him. Wrestling with these questions can motivate us to live God's way.

This section encourages young teens to take their questions to God, the source of answers, rather than holding them in and feeling guilty about them. Any question that is important to us is important to God.

At first glance, sessions 9 and 10 look very similar. But each deals with a different aspect of the problem of evil. Session 9 examines evil and pain caused by people who choose to disobey God. Session 10 examines suffering that has no clear cause. Though no one understands fully, session 10 presents several explanations for suffering and encourages youth to discover the answer that increases their understanding of God and encourages them to trust Him.

Sessions 11 and 12 examine some tough but crucial realities. Many times, no means yes to something even better. Realizing this can help young teens who are eager for independence to respect, honor, and enjoy God's guidelines. Session 12 replaces the myth of "happily ever after" with "life is worth the work."

These sessions may not be easy to teach because the questions are hard ones. But discussing them with your teens increases the chance that not only they, but you, will understand God better and trust Him more fully.

SESSION 9

WHY DOES A GOOD GOD ALLOW EVIL? (Deuteronomy 30:15-20; John 10:7-10)

KEY CONCEPT

Most of the evil in the world is caused by people who choose to disobey God.

MEETING THE NEED

This session responds to the following student questions:
- "How can a good God allow evil?"
- "Why doesn't God stop crime, war, and starvation?"
- "Why do people hurt each other in dating and friendship?"

SESSION GOALS

You will help each group member
1. explain the source of most evil,
2. recognize disobedient actions which contribute to specific evils in the world,
3. realize that he or she can choose to add to the evil or good in the world.

SPECIAL PREPARATION

_____ Bring extra Bibles, pencils, markers, large and small paper, masking tape, and chalk.
_____ Set up seven chairs or obtain six figures for "We're All in This Together."
_____ Prepare cards for "The Way to a Full Life."
_____ Prepare the signs for "The Source of Evil."
_____ Duplicate Workout Sheets #17 and #18. Cut #18 into cards.

BUILDING THE BODY

WE'RE ALL IN THIS TOGETHER

Set up seven chairs in a row. Enlist six people to sit in the chairs leaving the middle chair vacant, like this:

X X X ___ O O O

The goal is to change sides according to these rules:
1. X's move only to the right.
2. O's move only to the left.
3. You can move either one space, or jump only one person at a time.

The people not in chairs can coach those who are in the chairs. When the X's and O's reach an impasse, they start over. Solution: Keep X's and O's alternated throughout the process, e.g., two X's should not be sitting next to each other as the result of a jump, until near the end when sides are almost switched. The following is a sample solution showing diagrams of how chairs would look taking 16 turns to switch:

1. X X X _ O O O
2. X X _ X O O O
3. X X O X _ O O
4. X X O X O _ O
5. X X O _ O X O
6. X _ O X O X O
7. _ X O X O X O
8. O X _ X O X O
9. O X O X _ X O
10. O X O X O X _
11. O X O X O _ X
12. O X O _ O X X
13. O _ O X O X X
14. O O _ X O X X
15. O O O X _ X X
16. O O O _ X X X

After the X's and O's have successfully traded places, ask these questions:

How important was cooperation to the game? (Very!) **What would have happened if one person decided not to work with others?** (Would keep entire group from solution; would have frustrated many; would alienate himself from the group.) **When did the X's have to consider the needs of the O's in addition to their own, and vice versa?** (Throughout the game; each side had to alternate or no one could win.) **What would have happened if one person felt that his getting to the other side first was more important than anyone else getting there at all?** (No one could have made it.) **Who controlled the process? How did power affect the way things went?** (Depends on your group; encourage youth to share their observations.)

Explain: **This game is a picture of the way things are in the world. God placed us here and let us know the rules. But many have chosen not to play by those rules. Rather than turning to God to meet their needs, many people try to find happiness in power, selfishness, and superiority.** Ask: **What has been the result?** (Causes problems for everyone else, brings pain and suffering, neglects other people's needs.)

Alternate suggestion: If you have less than six youth, use six people figures borrowed from a preschooler in your church. Label them "X" and "O" written on masking tape.

LAUNCHING THE LESSON

WHY DOES GOD ALLOW IT?

To further illustrate the source of evil, ask: **Why does our good God allow so much evil and suffering?** After several people have responded, supplement with this information: **God is not the source of evil and suffering; people are. He doesn't inflict pain; people do. People choose to criticize, drive drunk, murder, steal, and grow fat while others starve. God has created us with the choice to obey Him or to disobey Him, to choose happiness or sadness. When we live our way rather than God's way, we automatically cause problems for ourselves or for someone else. He has chosen to give us freedom of choice and for the most part let our choices determine the natural results.**

Ask these questions and discuss:

- **Will God be upset with me for asking why He allows evil?**
- **Did God booby-trap the world so that when we do wrong we are punished?**
- **Why did God give us a choice if He knew we wouldn't use it right?**
- **How do the more complex evils, like famine, happen?**

As you discuss the questions, emphasize especially these points:

- **Asking God our questions demonstrates that we trust Him to have the answers, not that we're criticizing Him.**
- **No, God didn't booby-trap the world. He gave us the secrets to happiness.**
- **The ability to choose to love and to do right were worth the risk of choosing to hate and destroy. It's called free will. God knows we don't like to be forced to do anything. A lot of people use their freedom to create joy: friendship, marriage, unity, loyalty, understanding, laughter, devotion. None of that would be possible if we couldn't choose.**
- **The more complex evils started out as little sins. One or more people pooled their selfishness to cause great pain. They may not have meant to create pain, but they did it just the same. For example, industrialists sometimes use land in foreign countries to build factories. This land, formerly farmland, can now no longer be used to feed the people of that country. Famine and poverty result. They didn't mean to hurt anyone, but they did. We must learn to think about both the long- and short-range results of our actions.**

EXPLORING THE WORD

To discover the biblical basis for our understanding of evil in the world, search Deuteronomy 30:15-20 and John 10:7-10 in these ways.

STAND WHEN YOU FIND IT

Briefly introduce Deuteronomy: **The Book of Deuteronomy is Moses' review of the teachings of God. Chapter 30 is especially clear: God has offered and continues to offer His people a choice.** Direct youth to open their Bibles to Deuteronomy 30:15-20. Say: **I will read several statements. Stand when you find the verse that proves the statement true or that proves it false.** Call on the first person who stands to read the verse and tell whether the statement is true or false. NOTE: If one person tends to be consistently first, introduce a rule that no one may answer two questions in a row.

1. **God has set before us life and death.** (True, vv. 15, 19.)
2. **We can choose prosperity or destruction.** (True, vv. 15, 18.)
3. **God wants us to walk in His ways (obey Him), but He doesn't promise us anything for it.** (False; He promises life and blessing, v. 16.)
4. **Turning away from God results in disobedience.** (True, v. 17.)
5. **God never lets anyone be destroyed.** (False; if we want to choose actions that destroy us, He lets us, v. 18.)
6. **God hopes we will choose death.** (False; choose life, v. 19.)
7. **The source of life and happiness is the choices we make.** (False; the source is God, but we can choose Him, v. 20.)
8. **Listening to God results in life at its best.** (True, v. 20.)

Offer group members the option of calling out a truth from the passage for others to find. Emphasize: **Not choosing God brings destruction, which is another way to say evil, pain, and problems.**

Discuss: **If God promises such a great life, why do people ignore and disobey Him?** (People think obeying God will take away their fun and freedom; people don't trust God; disobeying God looks more exciting than obeying Him; people don't understand God.)

Explain: **Deuteronomy has pointed out that the choices you make determine how happy or miserable you will make yourself and others. Most evil starts with a problem: anger, jealousy, insecurity, or another problem. The person with the problem chooses a path from the problem that leads to evil or one that leads to good.**

WORKOUT SHEET

Distribute copies of Workout Sheet #17. Direct group members to follow the path to each evil and then to write in alternate paths that would lead to good.

Explain: **These paths are simplified for the sake of space, but they do give a basic idea of how evil and good develop.** Ask for volunteers to share their choices for each path to good. Possible solutions would be: (1) My friend's crop failed; mine did well; I'll share some of mine with him; I'll find other people who can help too; health. (2) I'm mad at my friend; I'll count to 10; I'll forgive her; I'll talk it out with her; healed friendship.

THE WAY TO A FULL LIFE

Ask: **How could you demonstrate that those who disobey God are missing out on the best in life?** After they have shared ideas, point out the words on cards which you have taped to the wall: ANYONE BUT JESUS, THIEVES, GATE, PASTURE, FULL, and JESUS. Say: **Choose one word**

and find in John 10:7-10 a message for those who disobey God. State the message using that word. Supplement discoveries with these sample messages: ANYONE BUT JESUS wants to steal your joy. Believers (sheep) recognize these THIEVES and know better than to pay attention to their lies. Jesus is the only GATE to the happiness you're looking for. Jesus is your PASTURE, which means you can come in to Him for understanding and strength to solve your problems. You're missing a FULL life without Jesus. JESUS' goal is your happiness.

Ask: **How would you explain the problem of evil in one sentence?** Encourage several to respond. Summarize with this definition: Because of sin in the world, people choose to disobey God and these wrong choices result in evil. Emphasize that this is a simple definition that doesn't do the problem justice, but it's a start at understanding why there is evil.

APPLYING THE TRUTH

WORKOUT SHEET

Explain: **The ways people cause evil are not always easy to recognize.** To give your group practice in recognizing the cause-and-effect principle of pain, duplicate Workout Sheet #18 and cut apart the matches on it. Keep the original as the key to the matches. Give each person one of these cards and say: **You have either a problem or a cause. Find the problem/cause that matches yours and then sit down with your partner. If you aren't sure of your match, ask me.**

When matches have been made, explain: **There are three categories of evil indicated by the three signs I am taping to the wall. Move with your partner to the sign which describes the category that caused your problem. The three categories are:**

YOUR DISOBEDIENCE	SOMEONE ELSE'S DISOBEDIENCE	MANY PEOPLE'S DISOBEDIENCE

Answers:
Problems caused directly by your disobedience:
- Running a traffic light results in a crash and a broken leg.
- Letting anger have its way results in injuring someone in a fight.
- Treating your boyfriend cruelly results in his breaking up with you.

Problems caused by someone else's disobedience:
- A jealous friend spreads a rumor that gives you a bad reputation.
- An assembly-line worker is careless in adjusting a new automobile's brakes. This causes the brakes to malfunction and a fatal car accident results.
- An angry man mugs your girlfriend and she must endure fear and a traumatic court appearance.

Problems caused by many people's disobedience:
- Businessmen take away farmland in another country to build a factory. This causes poverty.

- Kids who want acceptance by a gang perform acts of violence and vandalism.
- One race decides it is better than another, refusing to hire or live next to the other race. The rejected race suffers poverty and poor housing.

As you review each type, ask: **Does anyone have another example of each?** Allow plenty of opportunity to share.

If time allows, distribute slips of paper and say: **Write a problem, type of suffering, or example of evil on this slip of paper. You may use more than one.** Collect the slips and place them in an envelope. Draw one out at a time and call for group members to state possible ways people caused these problems. If youth include problems such as diseases or problems with unclear causes, explain that we will study these next week. Keep those slips until then.

SPREAD THE GOOD

Ask: **What can we do about the pain in the world?** Follow up responses with: **We can choose to do good ourselves, to spread a little of the good rather than the evil. What could one person do to spread good?**

Examples:

- "No, I really don't want to drink. I'm driving home tonight and I want to be sure we all get there safely."
- "Let's make this house we're building the strongest one on the block. These people we're helping can't afford sturdy materials, but we could probably get some of the rich company owners to donate them. If we're going to build them a house, let's do it right and safe!"
- "You know that boy from the children's home who comes to our church? Let's invite him to help us with the project. Maybe if he has something positive to do, he'll quit pestering everybody!"

Ask: **How might your doing good give others courage to do the same?** (Positive peer pressure.) **How does understanding how evil is caused keep us from contributing to evil?** (Knowing the results of our actions helps us decide wisely.) **What would encourage others to choose to obey God and quit hurting each other?** (Seeing how well it works in your life; seeing the pain caused by their disobedience.)

Encourage youth by saying: **You can influence others by every action and decision you make. Your lifestyle brings a little more good or a little more evil every day.** Call on a volunteer to reread Deuteronomy 30:19-20. Direct youth to shout in unison as loudly as they can: CHOOSE LIFE!

FORK IN THE ROAD

The choices we make can make the difference between good or evil in a situation. The progression of choices in the "paths" below show how selfishness can hurt others. But how could the same situations be turned around for good? Fill in the blanks in the alternate paths with choices that would end in good.

HEALTH

↑ [ ]

↑ [ ]

↑ **Mine did well.**

MY FRIEND'S CROP FAILED

↓ **Mine did well.**

↓ **But I need it all.**

↓ **Too bad for him.**

↓ **POVERTY**

HEALED FRIENDSHIP

↑ [ ]

↑ [ ]

↑ [ ]

I'M MAD AT MY FRIEND

↓ **I'll show her how it feels.**

↓ **I'll spread a rumor.**

↓ **I'll never talk to her again.**

↓ **END OF FRIENDSHIP**

If you get stuck, try inserting some of these problem-solvers that lead to good:

- ASKING FOR HELP
- LISTENING
- WEEPING WITH THOSE WHO WEEP
- RESPONDING TO NEED
- REJOICING WITH THOSE WHO REJOICE
- SHARING
- FINDING SOMEONE WHO CARES
- PRAYING
- SHOWING LOVE, JOY, PEACE, PATIENCE KINDNESS, GOODNESS, GENTLENESS, FAITHFULNESS, SELF-CONTROL
- RECOGNIZING YOUR FEELINGS
- COUNTING TO 10
- FORGIVING
- BEARING ANOTHER'S BURDEN
- TALKING
- COOPERATING

WORKOUT SHEET # 18

Matching Game

TEACHER: Cut apart these cards and distribute them to students for the first activity under "Applying the Truth."

You run a traffic light.	You crash and break your leg.
You let anger have its way.	You injure someone in a fight.
You treat your boyfriend cruelly.	He breaks up with you.
A jealous friend spreads a rumor.	You get a bad reputation.
An assembly-line worker is careless in adjusting a new automobile's brakes.	The brakes malfunction and a fatal car accident results.
An angry man mugs your girlfriend. He doesn't even know her.	She experiences fear and a traumatic court appearance.
Businessmen take away the farmland in another country to build a factory.	With no way to feed or support themselves, the people enter poverty.
Kids join a gang in order to be accepted.	They commit acts of violence and vandalism.
One race decides it is better than another.	They refuse to hire or live next to the other race. Poverty results.

SESSION 10

WHY DO BAD THINGS HAPPEN TO GOOD PEOPLE? (Matthew 5:45; John 9:1-3)

KEY CONCEPT

There's no easy answer to the question of suffering. Though we don't know why pain comes, we do know what to do once it's here.

MEETING THE NEED

This session will respond to the following student concerns:

- "Why do children suffer horrible illnesses and disabilities?"
- "Why do good people suffer while bad people seem to do fine?"
- "Why does God allow tornadoes, diseases, and birth defects?"

SESSION GOALS

You will help each group member

1. brainstorm possible reasons for unexplained suffering,
2. discover what to do with suffering once we have it,
3. pinpoint specific actions that help us through suffering.

SPECIAL PREPARATION

_____ Bring extra Bibles, pencils, markers, large and small paper, masking tape, and chalk.
_____ Bring foil for "The Shape of Suffering" option.
_____ Bring the problems listed during last week's "Applying the Truth" activity.
_____ Duplicate Workout Sheets #19 and #20.
_____ Make the posters for "If It's Me" and "If It's You."

BUILDING THE BODY

Try one or both of these options to start the session.

MOVE TO THE LEFT

Arrange the chairs in one large circle. Instruct youth: **Move one chair to the left if the statement I make about you is true. If there's already someone in that chair, sit in her lap!** Say several statements, such as:

Move to the left if you haven't done your homework yet today.
Move to the left if you eat ice cream in winter.
Move to the left if you brought your Bible to this study.
Move to the left if you've ever suffered.
Move to the left if you wonder why you have to suffer.

Say: **I heard a lot of groaning and suffering when people sat in your lap. Some of you may not have been in real pain, but you with six people in your lap probably were! But the suffering was short-lived, and if the right person was sitting in your lap, you probably enjoyed it! There's another kind of suffering that's not as easy or fun—the kind of suffering for which we don't understand the source or the reason. I'm talking about suffering that comes from debilitating diseases, handicaps, disasters, and more. The question of suffering is a hard one. But maybe, just maybe, once we get to heaven, the reason for this suffering will become as clear as the fun we had in this game.**

THE SHAPE OF SUFFERING

Give each person a piece of aluminum foil and direct them to shape it into "suffering." Explain: **There are no right or wrong answers to this activity. We are simply trying to give each other a clearer picture of suffering and what it means.** Be sure to shape your own piece of aluminum foil to share. For example, you could crinkle the foil and say, "Suffering gets me all in knots. It hurts and I don't know what to do about it." After about three minutes, call for volunteers to share what they shaped. Say something positive about each sculpture.

LAUNCHING THE LESSON

WHAT'S THE REASON?

Ask: **Who can tell me a story of human suffering? Limit your story to 60 seconds.** Write on the chalkboard a one-word summary of each. Possibilities include: cancer, multiple sclerosis, paralysis, mental retardation, unexpected death, tornado, disability, fire, birth defect, etc.

In the last session, youth listed problems of suffering and evil on slips of paper. If any they listed have no clear human cause, read them at this time and add them to the list.

Say: **It seems like some people get more pain than they deserve.** Use examples youth list to summarize. For example: **In the same month Roberta's dad died, she learned she had terminal cancer. The Stephens family lost their house to a tornado. Catherine has struggled with rheumatoid arthritis since she was a child. But the guy who sells drugs to elementary children stays perfectly healthy. Why do you think good people suffer?**

As group members call out their ideas, jot them down on individual slips of paper and display them in a row on the table or floor for use several times during this session. Supplement with these possibilities: Suffering brings good; sin causes suffering; suffering draws people to Jesus; suffering tests our faith; we just can't understand; suffering encourages us to depend on God; God gives suffering to those who can handle it; suffering gives God a chance to heal us; Satan sends suffering.

If group members have read chapter 10 in the student books, ask them which explanations make the most sense to them and why.

Explain: **No explanation for suffering makes sense to everyone. We don't really know why there are tornadoes, birth defects, or illnesses. What then is the answer?** After several have shared their ideas, say: **We don't really know. The same explanation that comforts one suffering Christian confuses and embitters another. In the midst of suffering, God, not an explanation, is what we need. Every Christian needs to find the explanation that makes the most sense and best enables him or her to trust God. An explanation can make perfect sense intellectually, but if it doesn't help us through our pain, it means little. As we continue to try to understand, we can keep trusting Him, knowing that we don't have to explain Him perfectly to trust Him.**

EXPLORING THE WORD

WORKOUT SHEET

Say: **Let's examine some Bible passages that help us know what to do with suffering. The Bible doesn't include a passage that says, "Thou shalt suffer because . . . ," but it does give plenty of advice for what to do with suffering once we have it. One believer explains that the real question is not "Why?" but "What now?"** Give each person a copy of Workout Sheet #19. Direct them: **Decode each puzzle to discover three messages that give the answer to the "What now?" of a person who suffers.**

Review the answers by calling on a different volunteer to decode each puzzle and read the accompanying verses. Then call for comments. Supplement ideas with these comments:

Look for joy when you have trials (James 1:2-4). (Many people are quick to quote Romans 8:28 and Genesis 50:20 to assure that God turns bad experiences into good ones. But the verses don't say the bad experiences turn to good; they say that God brings good out of the bad. Suffering is never fun, but good can come from it. When you find joy in the middle of suffering, you demonstrate that God is bigger than pain.)

Develop perseverance, character, and hope (Romans 5:3-5). (Let God work in you to bring these qualities. You'll grow to understand what really matters in life and the hope of no pain becomes precious. We know that our hopes will come true, if not on earth, in heaven.)

Depend on God's strength, not your own (Philippians 4:13, 19). (We need God to get us through the pain and know what to do with it. He is bigger than all the suffering and He's definitely on our side. He can help us make sense out of the mess.)

Close the discussion with this comment: **All questions have answers, and it's OK to seek the answers even if we don't fully find them until after death. Because the question is important to you, it's important to God. Let questions draw you closer to Him. Let Him teach you what to do while you try to understand why people suffer.**

STUDENT BOOK OPTION

If you have the student book, call on a volunteer to read the list of actions above "See for Yourself" (listed below). If you do not have the student book, overview these other actions we can do when we suffer:

- We keep on.
- We look beyond the pain to other joy.
- We overcome our limitations.
- We concentrate on what we can do.
- We keep asking questions.
- We continue to trust God.

WORKOUT SHEET

Explain: **In our struggle to understand suffering and explain it to people who suffer, Christians have come up with some pat answers. Even though they may be partly true, they usually do more harm than good.** Distribute Workout Sheet #20. Explain: **Christians who suffer disease or disability were interviewed to discover what people said to them. They then told which statements helped them and which made things worse. We'll call the helpful statements "loving," and the harmful statements "pat." Mark each of these statements "pat" or "loving." The Bible verses will help you decide.** You may want to give each person just two statements to look up so they can remember those two without being frustrated by reading so many statements. Overview the statements by calling for volunteers to share their responses and explain them. Supplement with these comments:

1. PAT: God hates suffering as much as we do, even though He sometimes allows it. God gave Satan permission to bring suffering to Job; He didn't bring it Himself (Job 1:8-12).
2. Can be PAT or LOVING depending on how it's said. God can work good from the evil that comes to us, but people don't want to be told that the suffering itself is good.
3. PAT: Matthew 5:45 explains that bad comes to good and bad people alike, as good comes to good and bad people alike. Jesus Himself said that suffering is not always the result of sin (John 9:3).

4. LOVING: People with long-lasting diseases or injuries comment constantly how much it helps for friends to ask them what they want. It might be as simple as bringing a magazine, washing a sweater, or listening. But it helps.
5. LOVING: Suffering Christians say it's incredibly hard to find people who will accept their sad emotions. Because Jesus cried, we know crying is OK. We need friends who will be sad with us.
6. PAT: God promises His strength to anyone who has problems (Philippians 4:13). He doesn't choose strong people to give problems to (Matthew 5:45). This statement makes people want to respond, "Maybe I should be a poorer parent; then my child wouldn't have to suffer."
7. LOVING: It's OK to feel sad, angry, and frustrated. Talking those feelings out helps more than denying them.
8. LOVING: Feeling with your friend helps him know that he matters to you. Jesus wept over the death of Lazarus, even though He knew Lazarus would soon be raised back to life.
9. PAT: A misinterpretation of Romans 8:28, this statement is an attempt to make the suffering seem not so bad. But the sufferer wants to respond, "Easy for you to say!" Most who say this wish their friend didn't have to suffer, so they wish it away with their words. But it helps more to acknowledge the suffering than deny it, to talk *about* the suffering rather than try to talk it *away*.
10. PAT: This makes suffering people feel like you're belittling their problem. "Sure, it could happen to anyone, but do you care that it happened to me?" These words can come across as a test: "If you were spiritual enough, you wouldn't be struggling!" It can make people feel guilty for suffering or for feeling angry about their suffering.
11. LOVING: Simply continuing to be a friend is the most loving response of all. Suffering Christians explain that the hardest thing about suffering is friends who stop spending time with them. Because the friends don't know what to say or do, they do nothing. Rather than feeling cared for, the suffering person feels deserted.

Close by stressing: **People who suffer, including ourselves, need love more than lectures. They don't need to hear, "This is why you're suffering," as much as, "This is why I love you." It's OK to say, "I don't understand," and "I wish you didn't have to go through this." Rather than "God has a reason," say, "I know God will help you through this." Keep this Workout Sheet for ideas of what to say when someone you love is hurting.**

APPLYING THE TRUTH

IF IT'S ME

Explain: **There are two times to respond to pain: (1) When it's you; (2) When it's a friend. Let's briefly explore both of these. When it's you you'll want to do three things that all start with "G."** Roll out the large paper on which you have written these three actions:

- **Go to God**
- **Grieve**
- **Get on with life**

Explain each briefly with words like these: **Because God is on your side**

and He has the power to help you, you'll want to *go to Him.* Talk with Him about your positive and negative feelings. Ask Him what you might learn through the experience. You'll need to *grieve* over what you've lost, whether it's good health or an ability. Let yourself feel sad about it. God will heal you. Then *get on with life.* Focus on what you can do, not what you can't. Enjoying the good things you have can make it easier to get through the pain.

Call on volunteers to share ways they've handled their own suffering. Explain that sharing both helpful and harmful ways they handled suffering in the past can help all of us manage future suffering better.

IF IT'S YOU

Explain: **If your friend is the one going through tragedy, your actions start with "Keep."** Roll out the paper with these three actions:

- **Keep quiet**
- **Keep listening**
- **Keep going**

As you write the three actions on the chalkboard, call for group members to share what they think these mean. Supplement their comments with:

One of our biggest blocks to helping a friend in pain is that we feel we must give all the answers. But we don't have to. When you *keep quiet* your friend has the opportunity to talk about what she needs to talk about. Your friend wants love, not answers. *Keep listening* even if she's mad at God, depressed, frustrated, and confused. God wants to know her feelings and does not condemn her for them. He's the one who can help her through them. *Keep going* even when you don't know what to say or do. Ask her: "How can I help you today?" "What needs doing?" Assure her that you care through your presence, through cards, through telling her what you like about her. As Galatians 6:2 and Romans 12:15 emphasize, we're here to share each other's burdens and hard times as well as happiness. Close by emphasizing: **No matter what you come to understand about the problem of pain, what really matters is, do you trust God? Every experience in our lives, either good or bad, can draw us closer to or farther from God. Let's let pain, as well as good, deepen our closeness to God.**

ADDITIONAL RESOURCES

If you or your young people want to read further on the problem of pain, consult these sources:

Good Grief by Granger Westburg, Fortress Press. Explains how grief can heal us. Grief is important not only for those who suffer but for those who love them.
Joni by Joni Eareckson (Tada), Zondervan. Tells the story of how Joni came to understand her accident and subsequent paralysis. The person who helped Joni understand her suffering was a teenager.
Where Is God When It Hurts? by Philip Yancey, Zondervan. Rich with stories of how real people with real pain came to understand their suffering.

WORKOUT SHEET # 19

PUZZLED BY PAIN

The Bible tells us how to handle suffering and hard times. The puzzles below give clues to messages based on Scripture. Decipher the messages and then look up the verses that go with them. A sample puzzle is done for you.

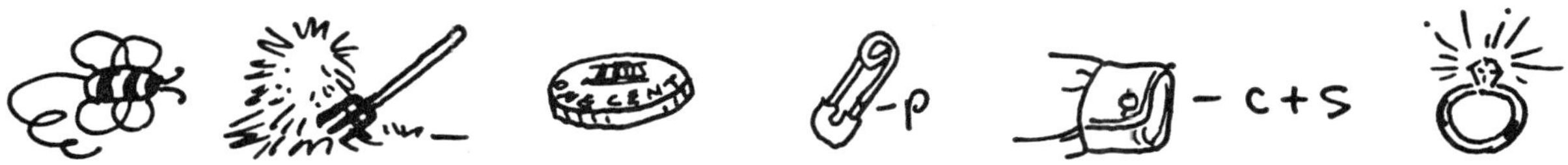

BEE (HAY-H+P)PAY CENT (PIN-P)IN (CUFF-C+S) SUFF RING

B E P A T I E N T I N S U F F E R I N G. James 5:7-11

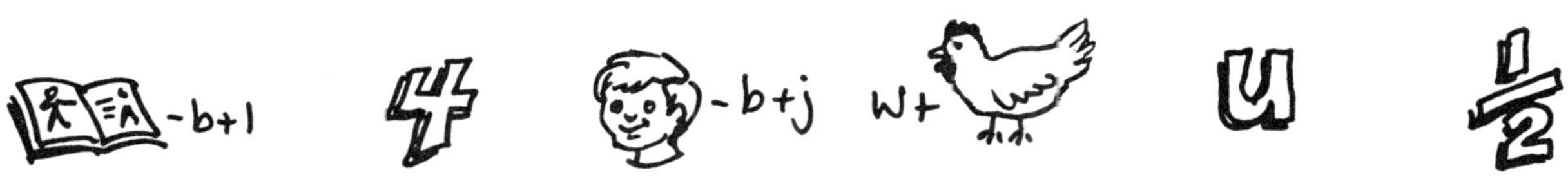

______ _____ _____ ______ ____ ______

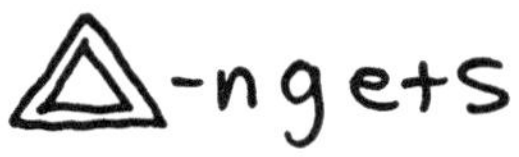

__________. James 1:2-4

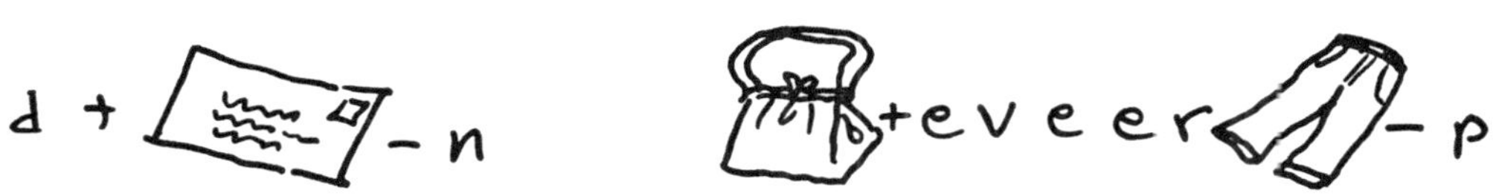

__________ ________________,

______________, _____ _______. Romans 5:3-5

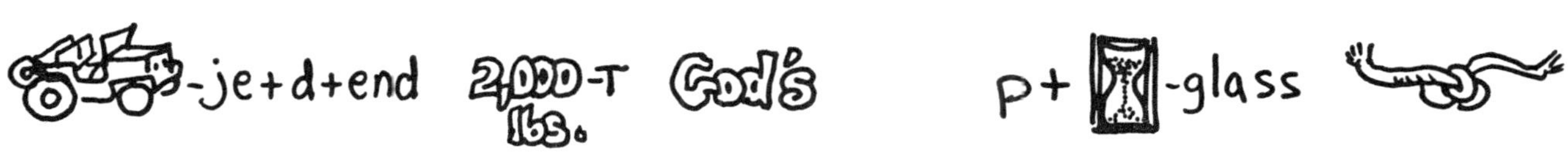

_________ ___ ______'__ _________, _____

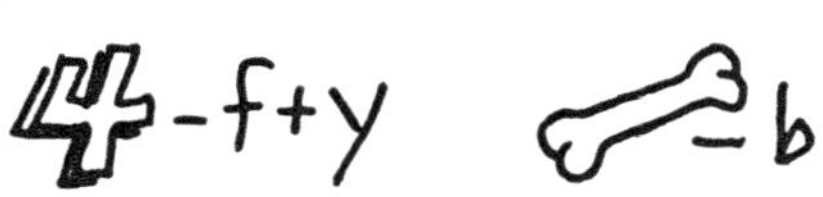

______ ______. Philippians 4:13, 19

NO MORE PAT ANSWERS

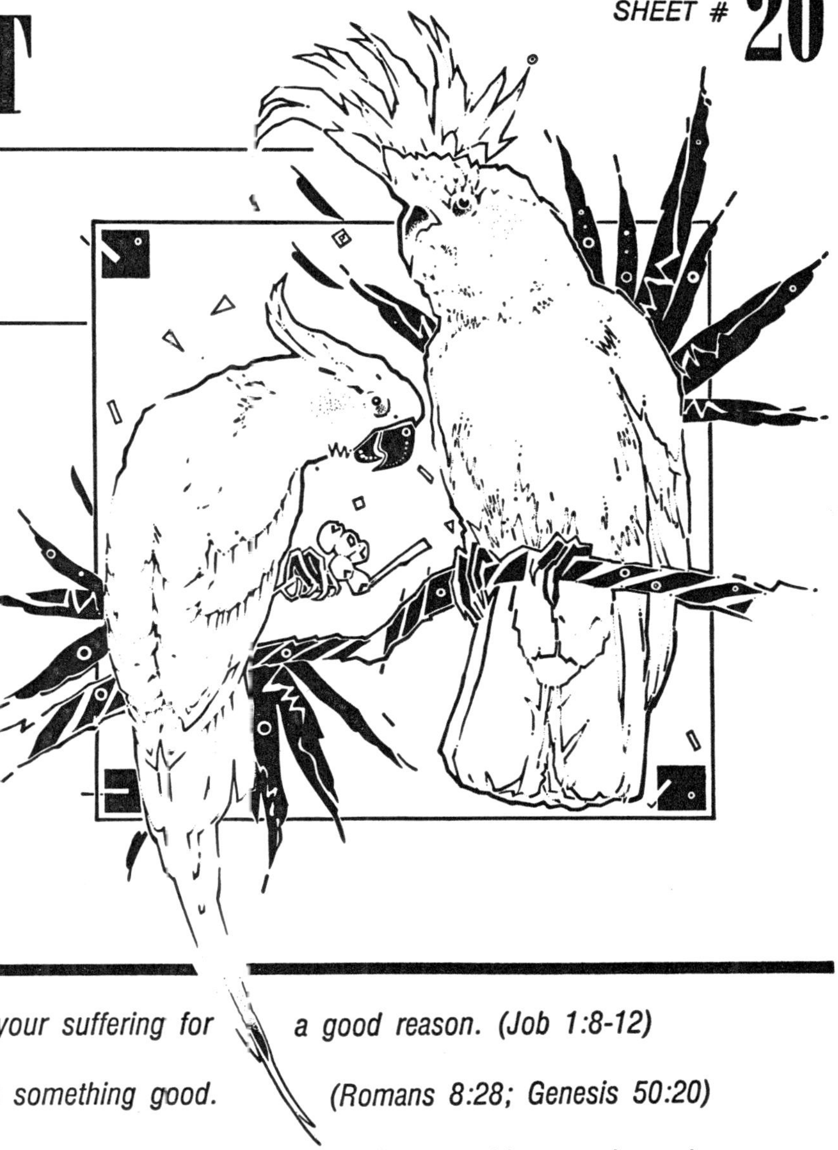

Have you ever had someone give you a pat answer that made you feel worse rather than better about your pain? A loving answer that shows the person cares is much better than a pat answer that's easy to parrot but doesn't do much good. Read the statements below and mark them Pat *or* Loving. *The Bible verses listed with them will help you decide by giving support for the statement or evidence against it.*

1. ______ *God must have caused your suffering for a good reason. (Job 1:8-12)*

2. ______ *Your suffering can bring something good. (Romans 8:28; Genesis 50:20)*

3. ______ *All suffering has a reason. God must be punishing you for something, maybe a sin you committed a long time ago. (Matthew 5:45; John 9:3)*

4. ______ *What can I do for you? (Galatians 6:2)*

5. ______ *It must hurt so much. Go ahead and cry. (Romans 12:15; John 11:32-35)*

6. ______ *God gave you a handicapped child because you're such good parents and He knew you could handle it. (Philippians 4:13; Matthew 5:45)*

7. ______ *I can see how you'd feel that way. (Romans 12:15; Job 16:15)*

8. ______ *I am so sorry this happened. (John 11:32-35)*

9. ______ *It's for the best. After all, it's not that bad. (Romans 8:28)*

10. ______ *It could happen to any of us. (Matthew 5:45)*

11. ______ *I care and I'm here whenever you need me. (1 Corinthians 13:4-8)*

SESSION 11

WHY DOES GOD SAY NO TO EVERYTHING FUN? (Selected passages)

KEY CONCEPT

God says yes much more often than He says no. His restrictions point us toward happiness; they don't destroy our fun.

MEETING THE NEED

This session will respond to the following student concerns:

- "I don't want to be a Christian because Christians never get to have any fun."
- "If I like it, God doesn't."
- "I know God said no. But He doesn't go to my school!"

SESSION GOALS

You will help each group member

1. picture fun as students at their school see it,
2. recognize the positive in God's restrictions,
3. stand up for God's view of fun.

SPECIAL PREPARATION

_____ Bring extra Bibles, pencils, markers, large and small paper, masking tape, and chalk.
_____ Bring the items for "Full or Empty?" or choose a confident youth for "How Heavy Is It?"
_____ Bring magazines, scissors, and glue for "Picture This."
_____ Duplicate Workout Sheets #21 and #22.
_____ Bring several translations of the Bible and dictionaries for "This Is the Life."
_____ Bring strips of paper for "His No Leads to Yes."
_____ Prepare the memorization cards for "A Verse Worth Remembering."

BUILDING THE BODY

Begin with one of these options.

FULL OR EMPTY?

Place on the table such items as a glass half full of water and math paper half completed. Ask: **What do you see?** Privately tally how many people say "half full" or "half finished" and how many say "half empty" or "half to go." Announce the tally and say: **There are two ways to look at these objects. Looking at the "empty" side can discourage us or even anger us. But looking at the "full" side can help us see the good in the situation.**

Ask: **Why does God say no to everything that's fun?** (A range of answers, probably including "to keep us from getting into trouble," "to show us a better fun," "to show us His way.") Ask: **How does the way we answer this question reflect how we view God?** Supplement comments with: **We can view God as wanting good for us or we can see what we are missing out on. Looking on the "full" side can demonstrate that what we're missing out on is something we don't want anyway, and what He offers is better!**

HOW HEAVY IS IT?

Choose a confident group member to assist you in this demonstration, and tell him or her the procedure ahead of time. Call this person to the center of the circle. Hand her a hymnbook, then another hymnbook, then another, and another until she starts to complain about the heaviness of the load. Say: **It doesn't look heavy to me. Here, take a couple more.** Keep adding hymnbooks until they fall. Ask the group: **Were the books heavy? How do you know?**

Supplement comments with: **The person actually holding the books knew more about how heavy they were than I did. I knew from my experience how many I could hold, but her capacity is different.** Ask: **How is God like the book holder?** (He's been through our experiences in the person of Christ. He also understands what we can take and not take because He created us. From our perspective we may think a certain action or attitude won't hurt us. But because God knows it will, He warns us in the Bible not to do it. We don't have to go through things to know if they will hurt us. We can depend on God to help us avoid a lot of pain.)

Ask: **How do you feel about God telling you not to do something?** (Probably both positive and negative.) After several have shared, say: **God has the best ideas for fun. Sin looks fun but deceives. It always brings pain.**

LAUNCHING THE LESSON

PICTURE THIS

Display colorful magazines, scissors, glue, markers, and large paper. Direct group members: **Choose a partner or two and get a large piece of paper. On that paper, write, draw, or attach pictures of fun as the people in your school see it. What do most young teens do on weekends? If your parents weren't home, what would you most want to do? Make a collage that depicts these types of fun.** Circulate and encourage the teams as they work.

Call for each team to hold up its collage and describe it. Instruct them to tape their collages to the wall after they've been presented. Challenge each team: **Choose one "fun" thing on your collage and tell what you think God thinks about it.** (Example: Drinking—He doesn't want us to get drunk; in the Old Testament, Levi took a vow not to drink at all.) **Why does God feel this way?** (Example: He doesn't want us to hurt ourselves or others.) **What are the dangers and pleasures of this type of fun?** (Example: Danger—drunk driver can kill someone on way home, can lead to alcoholism, even when you don't feel drunk you can be "out of touch." Pleasure—feels good.) **What might be an even more fun way of finding the same kind of pleasure?** (Telling jokes, games and challenges, acting silly but without drinking.)

Though many of the fun things may be negative, like drinking, drugs, and vandalism, be certain to focus on positive fun that we have. Emphasize the reasons God likes these kinds of fun. If they don't picture any positive, ask: **What positive fun do kids at your school have? What ways have you found to have positive fun?** (Talking with friends; goofing off together; going out in groups; eating; laughing.)

Explain: **God is the author of fun. He wants us to enjoy an exciting life, not suffer through a dull one. Why do you think He prohibits some "fun"?** (To protect us; to keep us from hurting ourselves or someone else.) **Why do these prohibited "fun" things seem fun anyway?** (Devil makes them look that way; are fun for awhile but backfire later.)

STUDENT BOOK OPTION

If you have the student books, call on someone to read the story about the cars in Anytown in chapter 11. Ask: **How are we like these cars?** (We want to do it our way; we get frustrated by rules.) **Why does it help to trust God's rules?** Just as the van didn't realize that the traffic rules and roads actually gave it more freedom, God's rules give us freedom to live a full life.

Emphasize: **God gives the rules to teach us about the way things work best. Rather than stopping our fun, they increase it!**

EXPLORING THE WORD

THIS IS THE LIFE

Explain: **Let's find out what kind of life God has in mind for us.** Call for a volunteer to read John 10:9-10 and another to read Jeremiah 29:11. Remind them that we studied John 10:7-10 in session 9. Review it by asking these questions:

- **To what does Jesus compare Himself?** (A gate, vv. 7, 9.)
- **Who are the sheep?** (Those who respond to Jesus by becoming Christians, vv. 7-9.)
- **What do the thieves want to do?** (*Steal* our joy, *kill* our happiness, *destroy* our relationships, v. 10.)
- **What do the sheep find when they go in and out of the gate?** (Pasture, v. 9.)
- **What might be our pasture?** (Whatever feeds and meets our needs, like friends, fun, challenges, ideas, help for problems.)

WORKOUT SHEET

Give each person a copy of Workout Sheet #21 and direct them: **Write what Jeremiah 29:11 means, in your own words, by simplifying each word or group of words. For example, "prosper" could become "succeed" or "become happy."** Provide several translations of the Bible and dictionaries to help. (Sample paraphrase: "God already knows the plans He has for me and they are good ones. He wants me to succeed and find safety. He won't hurt me. He wants me to have confidence about my tomorrows.")

Call for several to read their paraphrases. Emphasize, using the paraphrases: **God wants us to have the happiest life imaginable. That's why He lets us know how to find happiness.**

HIS NO LEADS TO YES

Invite youth: **Share about a time you said no to a friend or family member.** If they hesitate longer than a minute, share this example: "I told my friend not to date the boy who was asking her out because he wouldn't treat her right. She deserved better." As youth share their stories, ask each: **How was saying no the loving thing in your situation?** Contrast examples where no was the right thing with examples where no was the wrong thing to say. In your example, the loving thing was not wanting your friend hurt and wanting your friend to date someone who would treat her well. You wanted happiness for your friend, not frustration.

Explain: **God is like that. When He says no, it's an attempt to point us to happiness. To understand this better, let's find the yes behind each of the Ten Commandments. I will give each pair of you a commandment to rewrite without "no" or "not." You can use only positive commandments.** Direct them to turn to Exodus 20:1-17 and assign one commandment to each pair. If you have less than 20 in your group, assign more than one commandment to each pair or select the commandments you most want to emphasize. If you have more than 20, duplicate commandments. Give each team a strip of paper on which to write the positive command. As they complete commands, direct them to tape them to the wall in order.

This chart gives the verse reference and a sample paraphrase for each commandment.

1. Verse 3:	"Consider God more important than any other person or thing in your life."
2. Verses 4-6:	"When you worship idols, showing your affection to false gods, I feel jealous toward you rather than loving; and I want to show you love and make you happy."
3. Verse 7:	"Use My name in a way that makes Me look good and honors Me."
4. Verse 8:	"On Sunday rest from your usual activities and make it a day set apart for God."
5. Verse 12:	"When you honor your mother and father, you live longer (and are happier)."
6. Verse 13:	"Respect the life of every person."
7. Verse 14:	"Enjoy sex only with your spouse."
8. Verse 15:	"Take only what you have paid for."
9. Verse 16:	"Speak the truth about other people."
10. Verse 17:	"Be happy with what you have."

Review the commands youth have written. Compliment the group for their good work and precise insight. Ask: **What other commands of God seem like they take away our fun? Let's list them and find the positive to them.** As youth call them out, encourage the group to state each one positively. (Example: "Don't get drunk" in Ephesians 5:18-19 could be stated, "Have fun using your full senses, instead of with a dulled brain, and experience the full life the Holy Spirit offers.") Explain that they do not have to know the Scripture reference for the commandment. But be sure the commandments they state are biblical! Some "verses," like "God helps those who help themselves," are not in the Bible at all.

A VERSE WORTH REMEMBERING

Guide the group to memorize Jeremiah 29:11 by writing each word on a separate card, shuffling the cards, and putting the cards in order. To save time duplicate a copy of Workout Sheet #21 and cut it apart.

After youth have put the cards in correct order, read the verse in unison. Then say: **Now I will remove two words, and I want you to repeat the verse, filling in the two missing words.** Remove two more words, and repeat the process. Continue until all cards are removed and group members are saying the verse by memory. Ask: **What does this verse teach you about God's no's?** (He's on my side; He has plans to make me happy; because He has power to make His plans come true, I can trust Him to make me happy.) Encourage youth to repeat this verse whenever they doubt God's desire for their fun and happiness.

APPLYING THE TRUTH

DEVIL'S ADVOCATE

Pretend to be on the devil's side and try to convince your group that God really is out to spoil their fun. Say: **Your job is to prove me wrong. I'm convinced that God says no to everything and just doesn't want you to find out about the fun things.** Use comments like these:

- God won't let us have any fun parties. Everyone knows you have to drink and do drugs to have a good time. God just doesn't understand.
- God is for restrictions. Being your own boss brings real freedom!
- God doesn't understand that people won't like me if I don't have fun their way.
- God is always saying no to sex—no sex before marriage, no running around during marriage. He doesn't understand the current times. Let's enjoy the good gift He gave with as many people as possible!

If you have the student books, direct your group to scan chapter 11 for ways to defeat these arguments. If you do not have the student books, suggest that they recall points learned during this study. Hint that they might point out a positive for every negative you state.

OPPOSITES DON'T ATTRACT

Say: **Did you know that your will and God's will are not opposites? Name something you want that God also wants for you.** Challenge group members to come up with at least 25 areas of agreement, taking turns suggesting areas. Supplement with these: happiness, a good boyfriend/girlfriend (if not now, later), good relationship with parents, eventual independence, ability to make my own decisions, good grades, ability to understand homework, friends who like me as I am, job I enjoy.

WORKOUT SHEET

Distribute copies of Workout Sheet #22. Say: **Find the message by unscrambling the words.** When they have finished, check answers. (FOOD, PHONE, READ, REPORT CARDS, UGLY; decipher FODNEREADTCUG to make GOD CREATED FUN.) Say: **Sometimes it's hard for us to see the good when God says no. We want to do it our way. But just as it was worth the work to decipher this code, it's worth the effort to understand and live God's way.**

PLANS FOR MY FUTURE

WORKOUT SHEET #21

Write the following verse in your own words by substituting words that mean the same thing. For example, "prosper" can mean "succeed." Look at several Bible translations for ideas.

"For I know the plans I have for you," declares the Lord, "plans to prosper you and not to harm you, plans to give you a hope and a future." (Jeremiah 29:11)

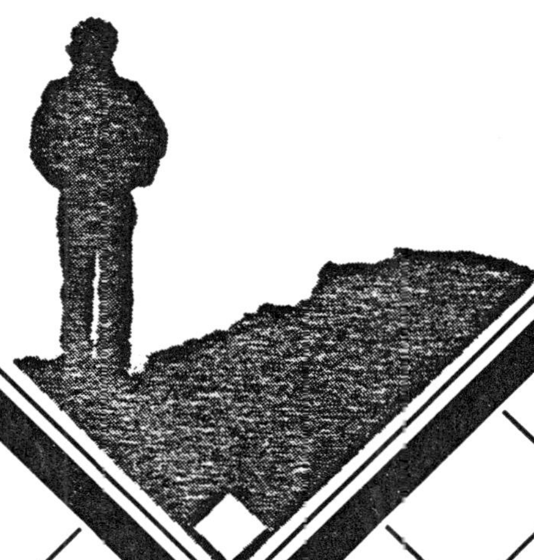

WHY TRUST HIM WHEN HE SAYS NO?

WORKOUT SHEET # 22

There's an excellent reason for finding out how to have fun God's way. Answer the questions and then arrange the circled letters to discover this reason.

◯ __ ◯◯

1. *We love to eat this when we get together.*

__ __ __ ◯◯

2. *We love to talk on this.*

◯◯◯◯

3. *We do this to books.*

__ __ __ __ __ ◯ ◯ __ __ __ __

4. *Schools send these home about every six weeks.*

◯◯ __ __

5. *When we're not feeling pretty, we feel ____.*

◯◯◯ ◯◯◯◯◯◯◯ ◯◯◯

WHAT'S OUR PROBLEM?

SESSION 12

WHY IS THE CHRISTIAN LIFE SO HARD? (Romans 7:15–8:2; Colossians 3:1-17)

KEY CONCEPT

The advantage of Christianity is not the absence of problems but the presence of help. Jesus makes life worth the work.

MEETING THE NEED

This session will respond to the following student concerns:

- "If God loves me, why is my life so hard?"
- "I thought Jesus would take away my problems."
- "Life seems harder, not easier, since I became a Christian."

SESSION GOALS

You will help each group member

1. brainstorm problems and reasons why Christians experience them,
2. discover ways Christ defeats the struggle with sin,
3. pinpoint reasons life is worth the work.

SPECIAL PREPARATION

_____ Bring extra Bibles, pencils, markers, large and small paper, masking tape, and chalk.
_____ Bring the items for "Miniature Olympics."
_____ Duplicate Workout Sheets #23 and #24.
_____ Duplicate the case studies.
_____ Write out the assignments for "Teamwork."

BUILDING THE BODY

Begin the session with one of these openers.

MINIATURE OLYMPICS

Play several mini-olympic games, such as javelin throw (with drinking straws) and 50-yard dash (whoever draws 50 dashes first wins).

Discuss the experience with these questions: **How difficult were these challenges?** (Pretty hard because we hadn't tried them before.) **Did you enjoy them?** (Answers will vary.) **What made the experience worth the effort, even when your effort did not pay off?** (Was fun, challenging, enjoyed playing with friends.)

Explain: **Most difficult experiences have results that make them worth the work. It's the same way in Christianity. Let's find out why.**

GLAD TO BE A CHRISTIAN

Instruct group members to stand in one big circle and each call out a reason he or she is glad to be a Christian. No one may give an answer already given. When someone cannot think of a reason, he sits down. Stress that the reasons can be simple and short. Continue listing reasons until no one is standing. Pray, thanking God for all these advantages of Christianity.

Explain: **Christianity doesn't abolish our problems. In fact, it may create some. But the advantages of Christianity far outweigh the problems.**

LAUNCHING THE LESSON

A ROUND OF PROBLEMS

Arrange the chairs in one large circle. Give these instructions: **The person on my left will say her name and a difficulty that starts with the same letter or sound as her first name. The person on her left will repeat her name and problem and then state his own name and problem. For example: "Her name is *Jessica* and she finds *jealousy* hard. My name is *Karl* and one thing I find hard about life is I *kan't* pass my algebra tests." Note that Karl's problem started with the same sound and Jessica's with the same letter. The next person repeats both those before her and so on until the final person repeats everyone's names and difficulties. No two people can list the same difficulty.**

After this activity, signal someone you have previously enlisted to stand and say: "Wait a minute! I thought we were all Christians! If the Christian life is easier, why do we still have problems?" Call for responses to this question. Jot ideas down on large paper or a chalkboard.

Explain: **Problems are a part of life. The advantage of Christianity is not getting rid of our problems, but finding a Person, Jesus Christ, who can help us with them. Now instead of the problems defeating us, we can defeat the problems. During this session, we'll explore how.**

TWO KINDS OF PROBLEMS

Explain: **Problems come in two varieties: (1) Some come to everybody, Christian or not. What are some of these?** (Frustrations, relationship problems, unfairness, sadness, disappointment.) **(2) Some struggles come because of our commitment to Christ. What are some of these?** (Fighting temptation, trying to obey God when we don't feel like it, being laughed at for our faith.) Say: **Because we've spent 11 sessions focusing on the first type, we'll focus on this second type today. Even though it's hard to live the Christian life, the benefits are well worth it. As athletes say, "No pain, no gain."**

EXPLORING THE WORD

WORKOUT SHEET

Give each person a copy of Workout Sheet #23. Give these instructions: **You who have birthdays from January through June read the boldface lines and you who have birthdays from July through December read the light lines. Stand while you read your lines.** (Though they may complain about it, young teens enjoy the constant standing and sitting. It also demonstrates the up and down struggle to do right.)

Discuss the responsive reading with these questions and comments: **Your text came from Romans 7:15–8:2. Who can summarize the struggle in one or two sentences?** Encourage more than one person to give a summary. Each will bring out a slightly different but equally important point. (Sample: It describes Paul's struggle between doing what God wants him to do and what his old sinful nature wants to do.)

Say: **Notice the title of the Workout Sheet. Paul wants to follow Jesus. But his old sin nature or human nature makes it hard. How are our struggles like and not like this one?** (We all struggle with doing right and wrong; we don't always recognize a struggle with sin; rather than feeling like prisoners, we may just feel sad.)

Ask: **What does Paul say is the solution to our struggle?** (Freedom through Jesus Christ. He gives us the power to overcome anything that keeps us from obeying God.) **Why do you think Paul struggled so hard if he knew God's way is right?** Encourage several people to share their ideas and then supplement with these comments: **Some Christians call this "original sin" and others call it our "human nature." Whatever it's called, we humans are naturally rebellious. We want to do it our way, even though we know that God's way will make us happier. Knowing this battle is there helps us know how to fight it.**

Encourage your students to share a time they struggled between doing right and wrong. Ask such questions as: **What was so hard about it? What were the results of your struggle? What did you learn about yourself and about God?** Assure them that we all struggle to do right and that we can all encourage each other.

Ask: **What would happen if we quit struggling and just lived the way we felt like living?** (We'd find even more unhappiness; we'd create problems for ourselves.)

Ask: **What was it that helped Paul with his struggle?** (Realizing that Jesus had already won and had set him free.) Point out: **Happiness in life is a choice. We choose to live God's way and to enjoy the benefits of life with Him. Each time we struggle to do the right thing, we recognize a benefit of life with God. The next time the struggle might not be so hard. Learning to live God's way is like a cycle that becomes a very good habit: each time we live His way, we realize His way works, which makes us trust Him more, which encourages us to live His way. Colossians 3 suggests some specific actions to begin the habit of living God's way.**

WORKOUT SHEET

As you distribute Workout Sheet #24, instruct group members: **Separate the characteristics of freedom in Christ from the characteristics that enslave us. In this passage the enslaving characteristics are called "earthly nature" or "old self" characteristics. The freeing characteristics are called virtues or "new self" characteristics. Put the freedom characteristics on the Christian and the enslaving characteristics in the trash can.**

Call for volunteers to read the characteristics of the Christian and the characteristics they discarded. (Answers from the NIV translation [others will vary slightly]: *Earthly nature*—sexual immorality, impurity, lust, evil desires, greed, idolatry, anger, rage, malice, slander, filthy language, lying. *New self*—compassion, kindness, humility, gentleness, patience, bear with each other, forgive grievances, love, unity, peace, thankfulness, word of Christ dwells in you, wisdom, singing, gratitude, do all in the name of the Lord Jesus, giving thanks.)

APPLYING THE TRUTH

CASE STUDIES

Explain: **The battle to do God's will is not an easy one, but it's worth the work. "Happily ever after" happens in fairy tales, not real life. To discover the benefits of obeying God even when it's hard, we're going to use the freedom in Christ characteristics from Colossians 3 to solve these case studies.** Display the following case studies, one per pair of young people. **Choose a partner and a case study. Prepare to dramatize your solution to the situation and to answer the questions.** Explain that some pairs will have the same case study but that their solutions may differ. Encourage them to keep Colossians 3 open before them and to refer to Workout Sheet #24.

The case studies:

For several years Pam's parents refused to have anything to do with church or Christianity. They said Pam would outgrow her commitment when she learned to think for herself. Pam has tried to maintain respect for her parents even though she knows that Christianity is for people of all ages. Lately her mom has become more open to talking about Christianity, but still wants nothing to do with church.

1. How do you think Pam's *gentleness* and *patience* have opened her mom up to Christianity?
2. What other Colossians 3 characteristics in Pam might encourage her mom to become a Christian?
3. What helped Pam get through the years when her mom constantly criticized her faith?
4. What benefits, both now and in the future, made Pam's struggle worth it?

Luis practiced all summer for the ball team. Everyone who watched him complimented his ability. Luis felt confident, but not cocky, during tryouts. He had high hopes of making it. He made it past the first cut but was cut the second time. He was crushed. "Why? Why me?" he asked. That night at church he talked with Bill, a friend who had also been cut from the team. "Maybe we'll make it next year," Bill said. "Not many seventh-graders make the team."

1. How did Bill's *compassion* help Luis? What difference did it make that Bill had been through the same experience?
2. What other Colossians 3 qualities could help Luis and his friend through their disappointment?
3. What was hard about this situation?
4. What benefits, both now and in the future, could make Luis' struggle worth it?

Jan and Lori had been best friends for years. But now that they had reached junior high, things were changing. Lori wanted to be in the popular group and ignored Jan around them. Jan understood Lori's desire to be liked, but she didn't understand why Lori ignored her.

1. How did *forgiveness* help Jan continue to love Lori?
2. What other Colossians 3 virtues could help Jan and Lori work out this problem in their friendship?
3. What is hard about this situation?
4. What benefits, both now and in the future, will make working out this problem worth the work?

TEAMWORK

Explain: **Everyone's life has its difficulties and problems. The advantage of living God's way is that He is on our side to give us power and ideas for solving our problems. To demonstrate this, choose one of these teams.** Read each assignment and encourage youth to choose one.

REFEREES: Write a sports manual for the game of Christian living. Include the name of the coach, rules for play, fouls and penalties, and exercises that strengthen playing ability.

ADVERTISING CREW: Create a slogan and banner which shows why the Christian life is worth the work.

SPORTS REPORTERS: Write a newspaper story of "Junior High MVC" (Most Valuable Christian). Tell how this person handles his or her problems with the power of Christ.

RADIO/TELEVISION COMMERCIAL: Using the tune of a currently popular television or radio commercial, write a commercial encouraging people to let God help them solve their problems.

Call for the teams to present their creations. Congratulate each. Explain: **Through this activity, you have pinpointed reasons you're glad to be Christians and have highlighted advantages of Christianity.** Encourage them to live what they have said!

WHY NOT LIVE THE EASY WAY?

Write this letter on the chalkboard or large paper and direct youth to write an answer to the author of this paragraph:

> If the Christian life is a struggle, why be a Christian at all? Why not just live the easy way? Without God you don't have to worry about guilt, temptation, or obedience. You can be your own boss, make your own decisions, determine your own fate. I'd rather not struggle.
>
> No Work for Me!

Call for several people to read their responses. (Supplement with: Though life with God can be hard, life without Him is harder; being your own boss is not as easy as it seems; life is too complicated to go it alone; I want to spend my life in heaven, not hell; because God knows the secrets to happiness, it is worth following Him; God didn't give us the problems—He gives us the answers; God's way may be hard, but it's happier.)

PROBLEMS ARE A PART OF LIFE

Pray, thanking God for His problem-solving power. Try one or more of these options. Ask group members to . . .

- Call out a problem God has helped them solve.
- Call out a quality they love about God.
- Praise God for a way they've seen His power demonstrated.

To close the session and this study, reemphasize: **Having problems does not mean you're bad or weird. It means you're human. As a Christian you have a definite advantage because you're in touch with the Problem-solver. Attack each problem as it comes and concentrate on the joy. Rather than letting problems get you down, let them get you growing. You and God can solve anything that comes along.**

WHY CAN'T I DO WHAT I WANT TO DO?

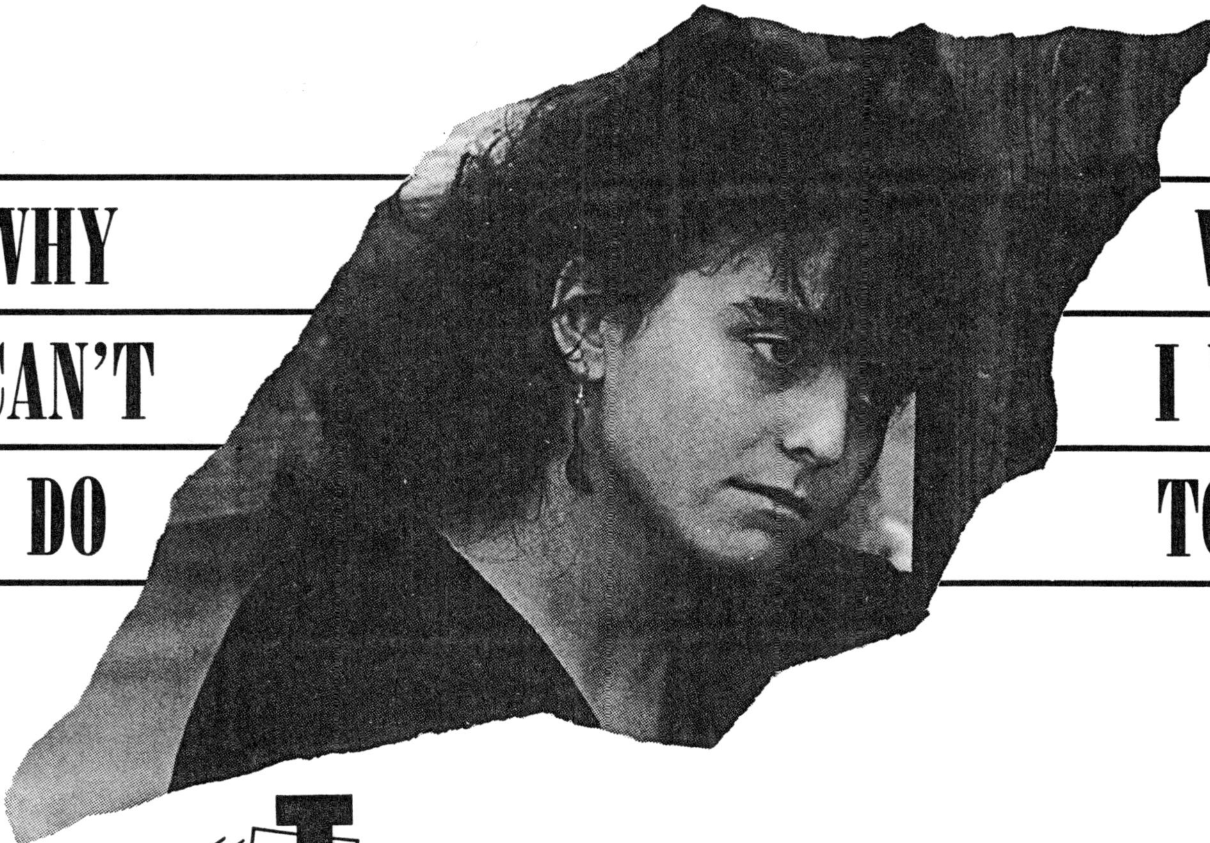

This responsive reading is from Romans 7:15–8:2. In it Paul shares the struggle he has trying to do right.

I do not understand what I do.
For what I want to do I do not do, but what I hate I do.
And if I do what I do not want to do, I agree that the law is good.
As it is, it is no longer I myself who do it, but it is sin living in me.
I know that nothing good lives in me, that is, in my sinful nature.
For I have the desire to do what is good, but I cannot carry it out.
For what I do is not the good I want to do;
no, the evil I do not want to do—this I keep on doing.
Now if I do what I do not want to do, it is no longer I who do it, but it is sin living in me that does it.
So I find this law at work:
When I want to do good, evil is right there with me.
For in my inner being I delight in God's law;
but I see another law at work in the members of my body, waging war against the law of my mind.
and making me a prisoner of the law of sin at work within my members.
What a wretched man I am!
Who will rescue me from this body of death?
Thanks be to God—through Jesus Christ our Lord!
So then, I myself in my mind am a slave to God's law,
but in the sinful nature a slave to the law of sin.
Therefore, there is now no condemnation for those who are in Christ Jesus,
because through Christ Jesus the law of the Spirit of life set me free from the law of sin and death.
Romans 7:15–8:2

HAPPINESS IS A *Choice*

WORKOUT SHEET # 24

Happiness seldom comes easily, but it always comes to those who are willing to live out their commitment to Jesus Christ. Search Colossians 3:1-17 for characteristics you want to develop and some you want to discard. The "rejects" are called "earthly nature," so they belong in the trash. Write them there. The "new self" qualities belong on the Christian, so write them there.

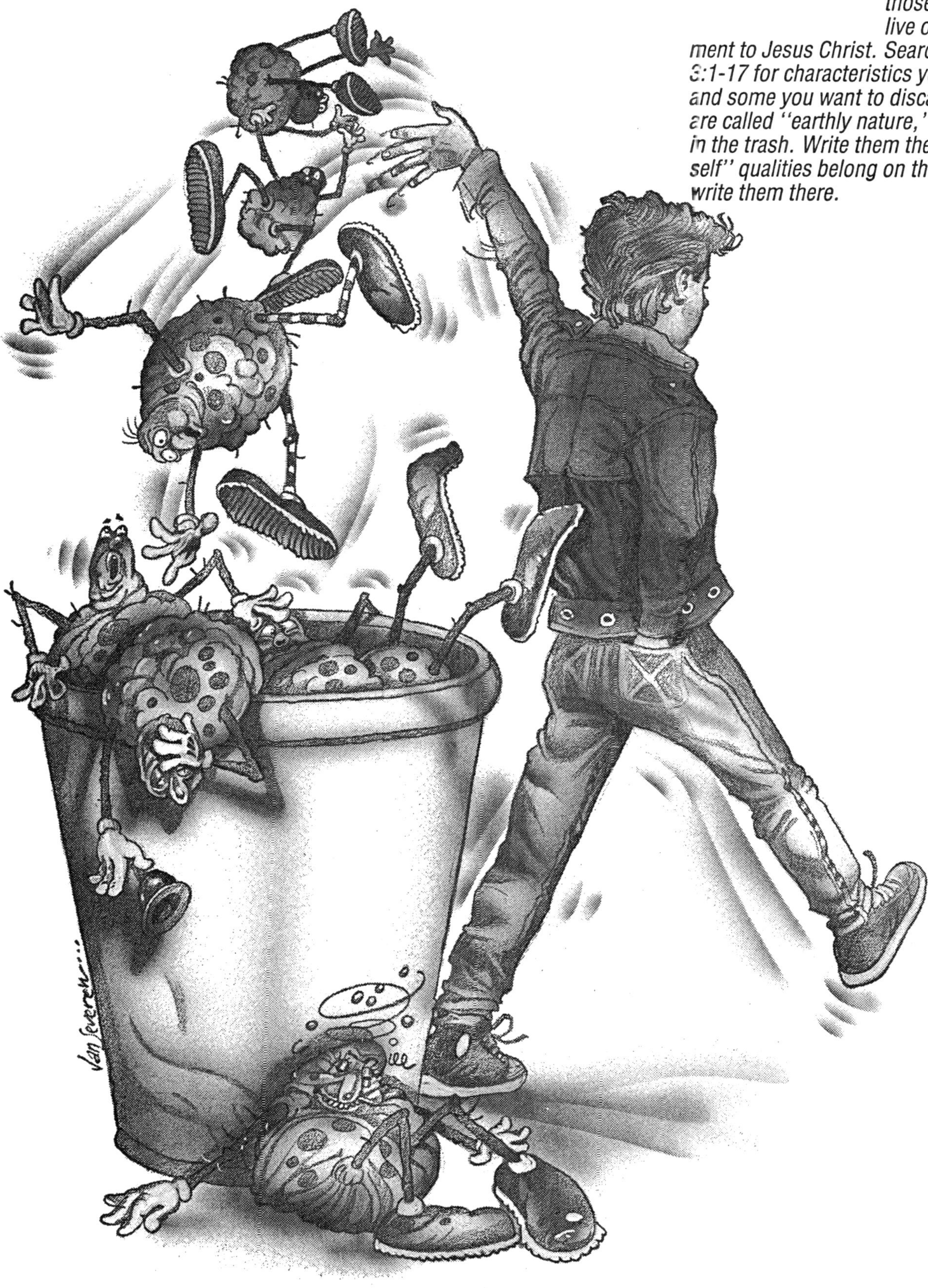

WHAT'S YOUR PROBLEM?

EVALUATION SHEET

Dear Leader,

You can have a real impact on future Young Teen Feedback Electives! Please take a minute to fill out this form giving us your candid reaction to this material. Thanks for your help.

ABOUT YOU

In what setting did you use this elective? (Sunday School, youth group, midweek Bible study, etc.)

___

How many young people were in your group? ______

What was the age-range of those in your group? ______

How many weeks did you spend on this study? ______

How long was your average meeting time? ______

(Optional) Name ______

Address ______

ABOUT THIS YOUNG TEEN FEEDBACK ELECTIVE

Did you and your young people enjoy this study? (Why or why not?)

What are the strengths and weaknesses of this leader's book?

Did you use the student books? ______ Yes ______ No

If so, what are their strengths and weaknesses?

ABOUT THE FUTURE

What topics and issues would you like to see covered in future electives?

What Bible studies would you like to see included in future electives?

Do you plan to use other Young Teen Feedback Electives? (Why or why not?)

Do you plan to repeat this study in the future with new students? (Why or why not?)

Place
stamp
here

SonPower Youth Sources Editor
1825 College Avenue
Wheaton, Illinois 60187